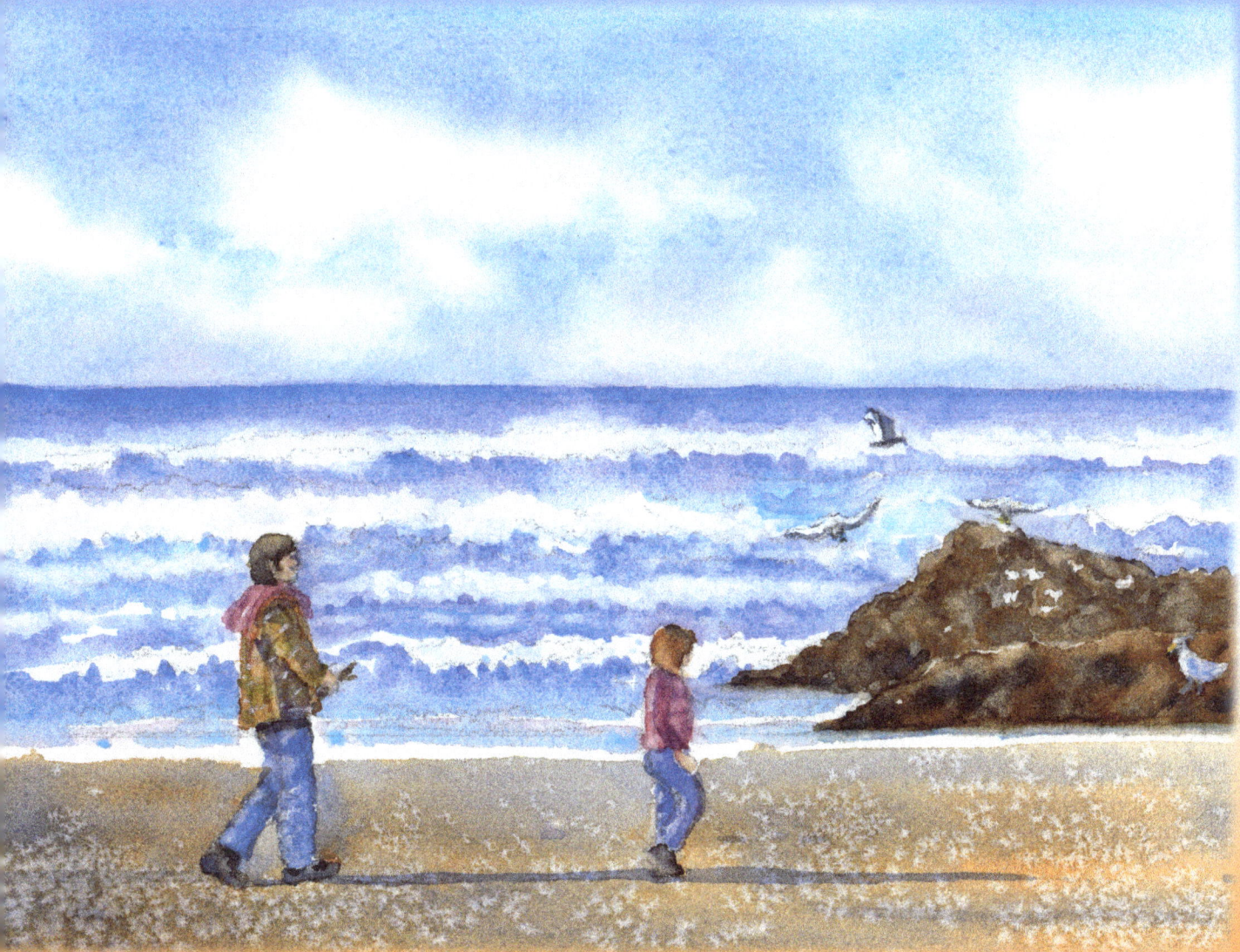

The Wind In Me

Thank you to
C.W. Smith &
Frank Gonzalez

For Noah, Ethan, Joshua,
Isabella, Olivia and
all of the children of the world.

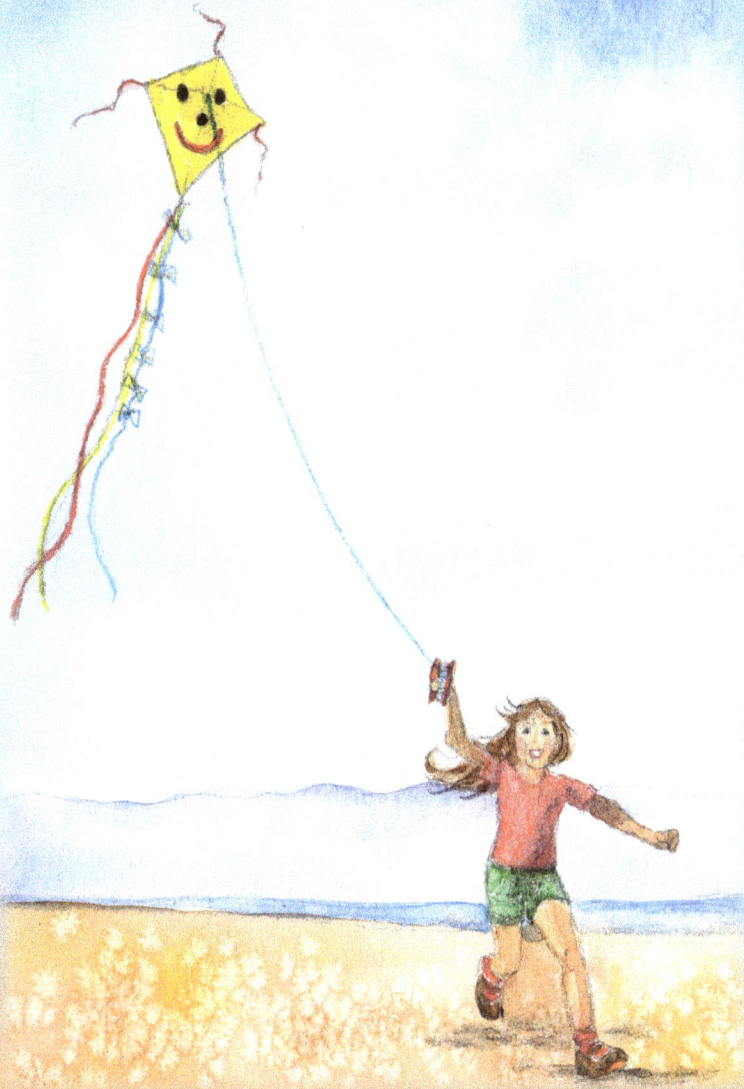

The Wind In Me
The first step in sensing your bodymind.

By Diane Smalley

Illustrated by Ann Meyer Maglinte

Everyone

breathes.

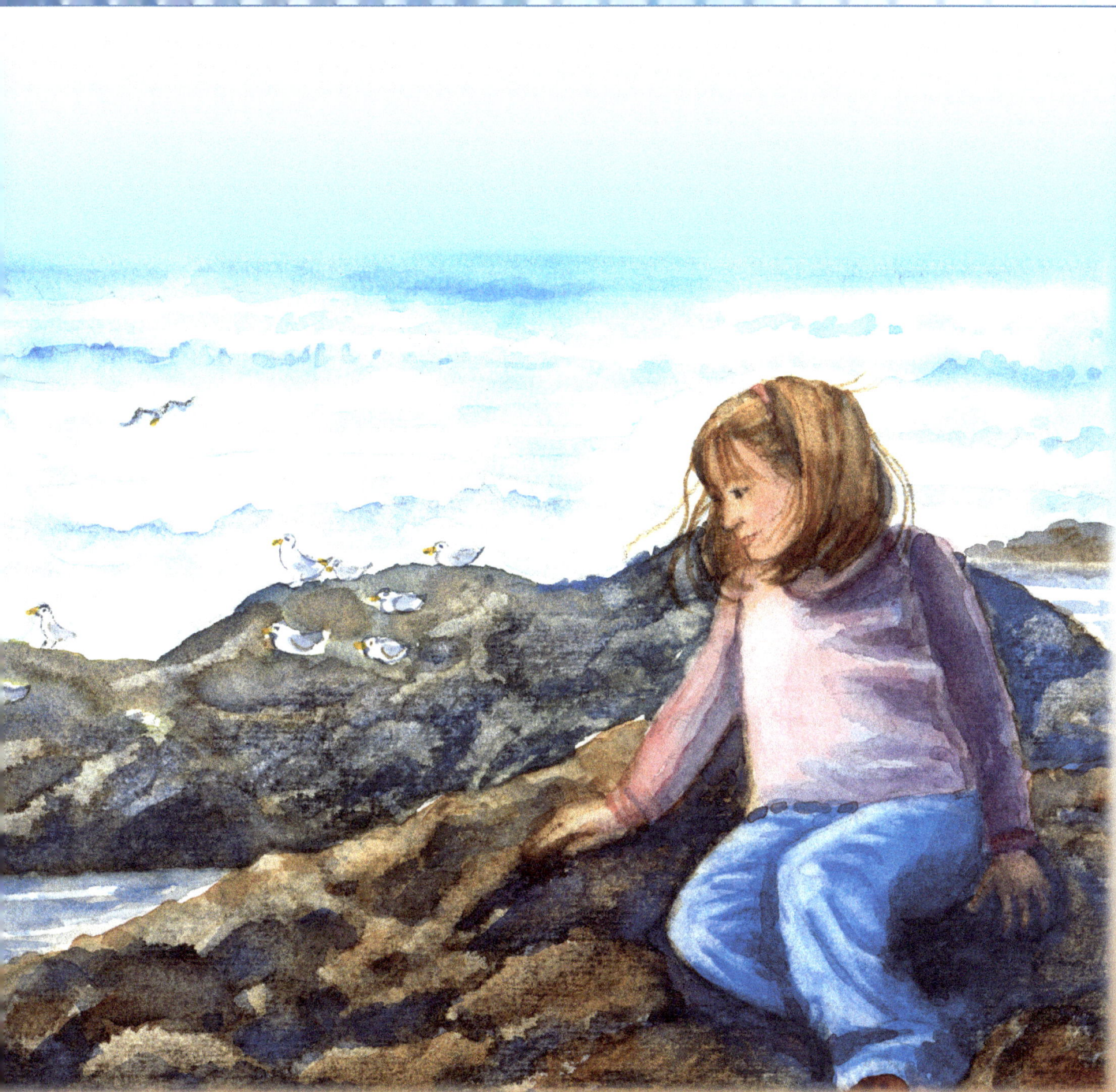

Some
beings
breathe
very
slowly.

A tree
takes a
whole
day
for one
breath!

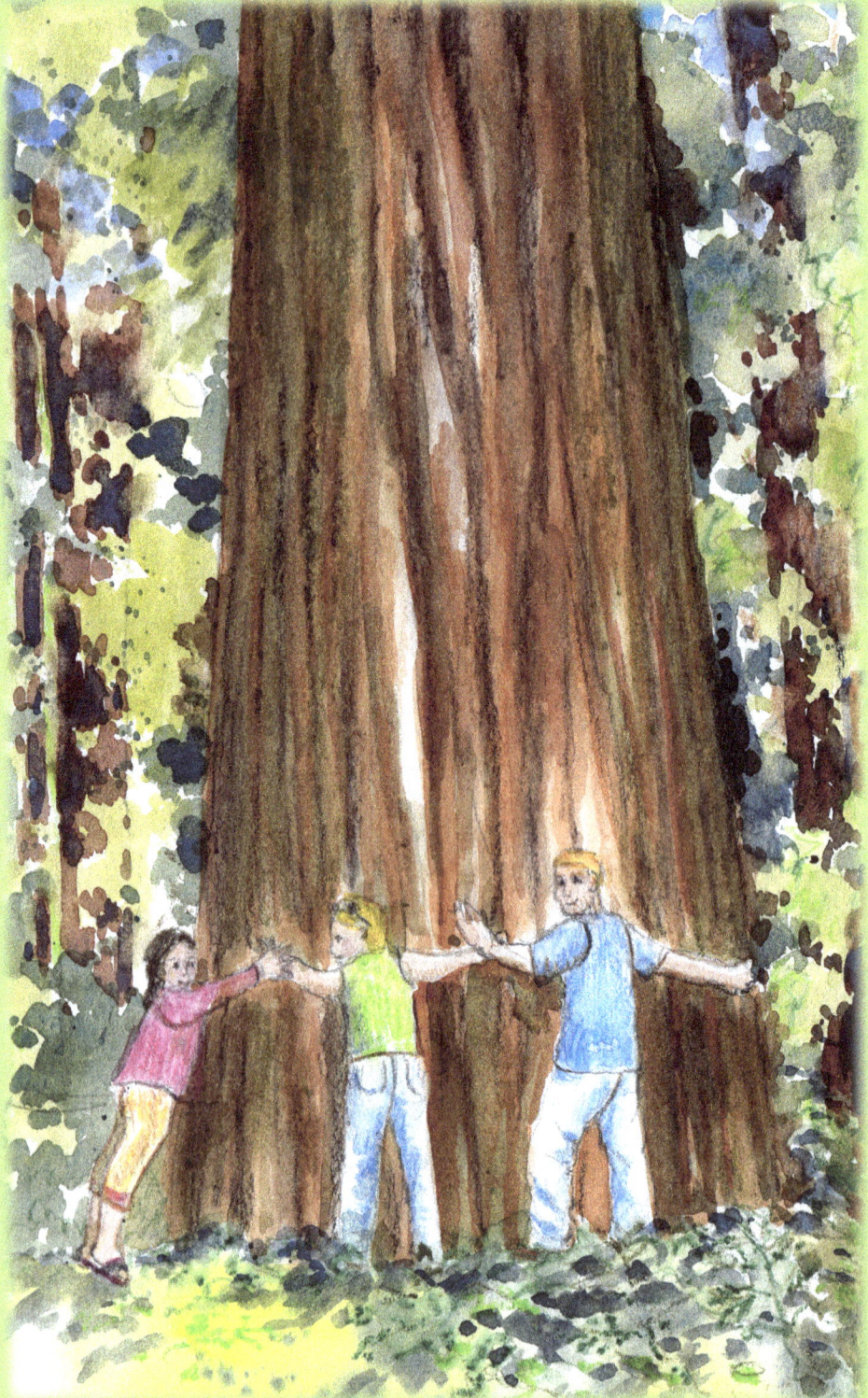

Some beings breathe very fast.

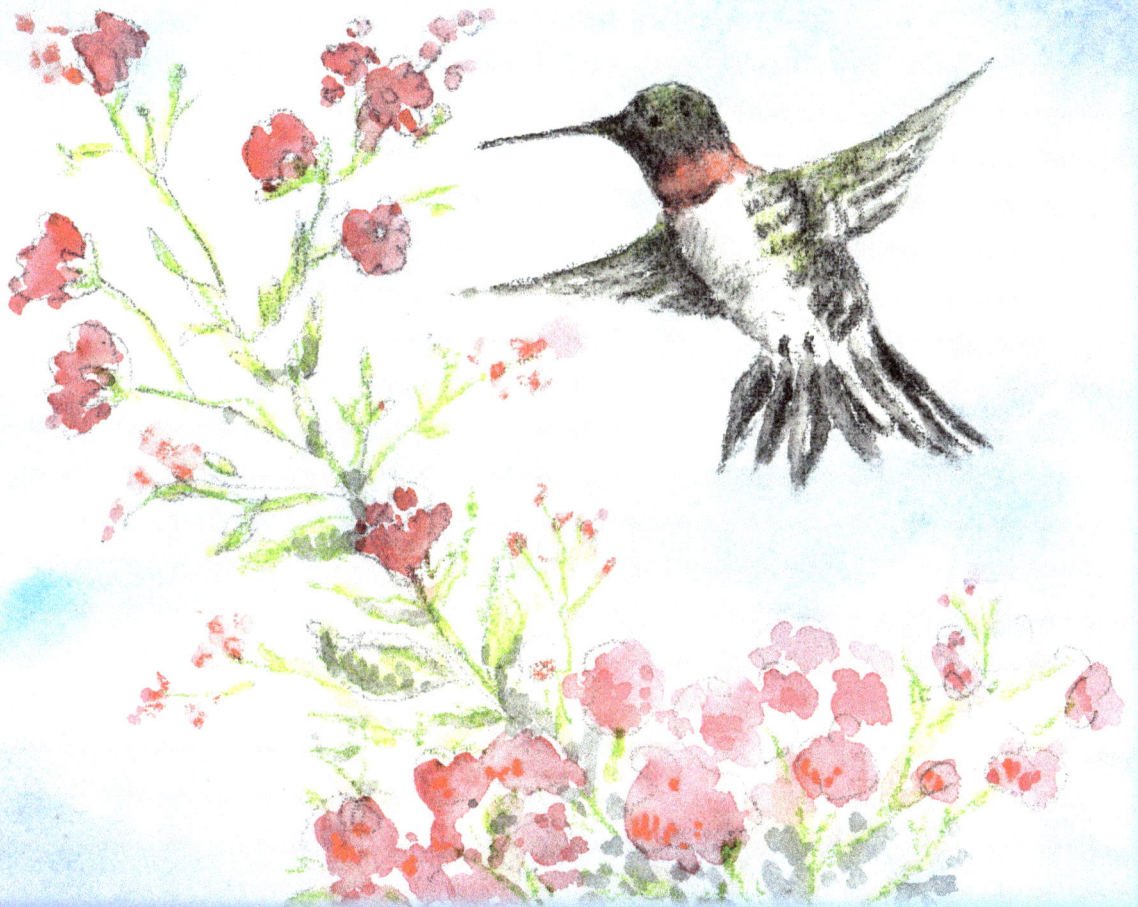

A hummingbird takes 250 to 1200
breaths each minute!

My breath has a rhythm that is

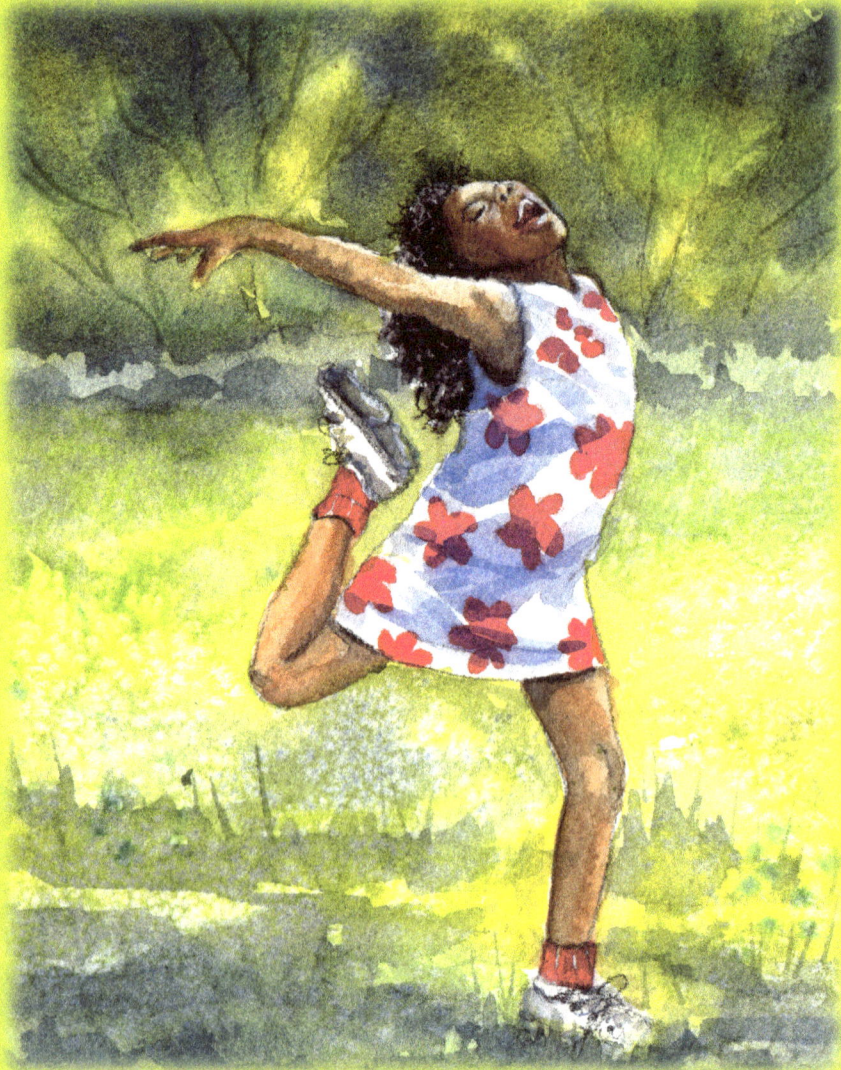

just right for me.

The wind in me gives me life.

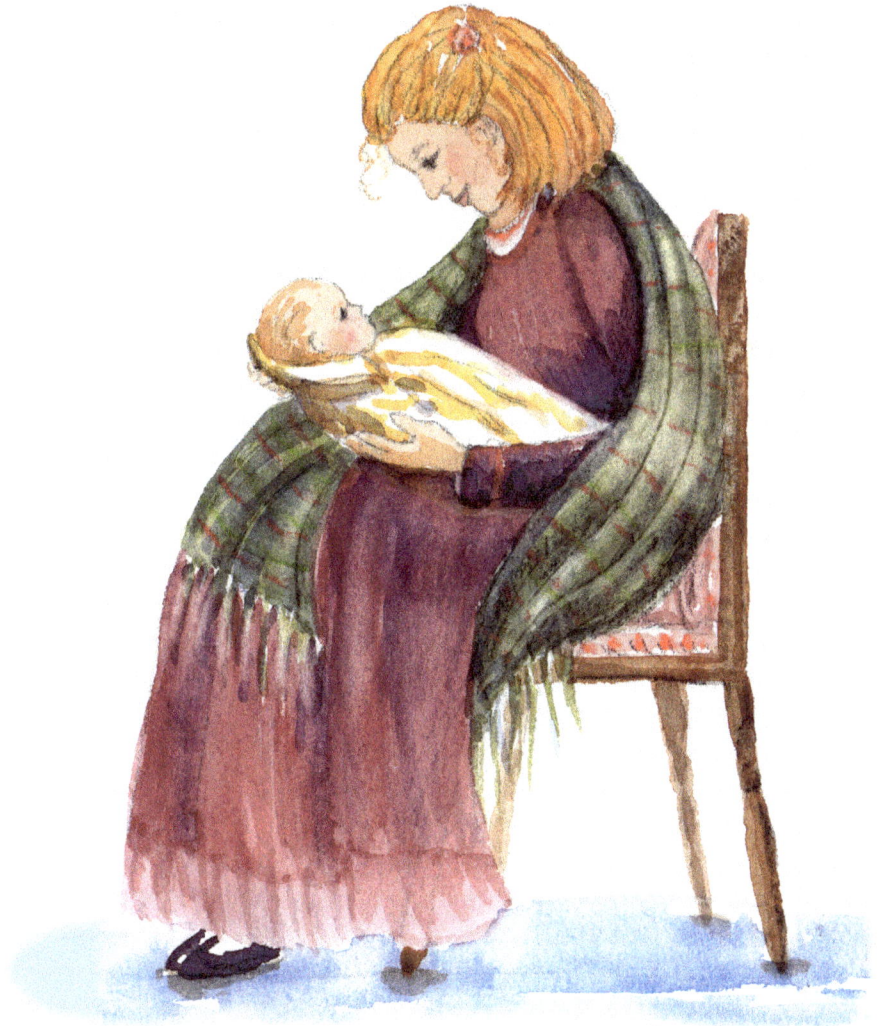

My breath happens when
I am not noticing it…

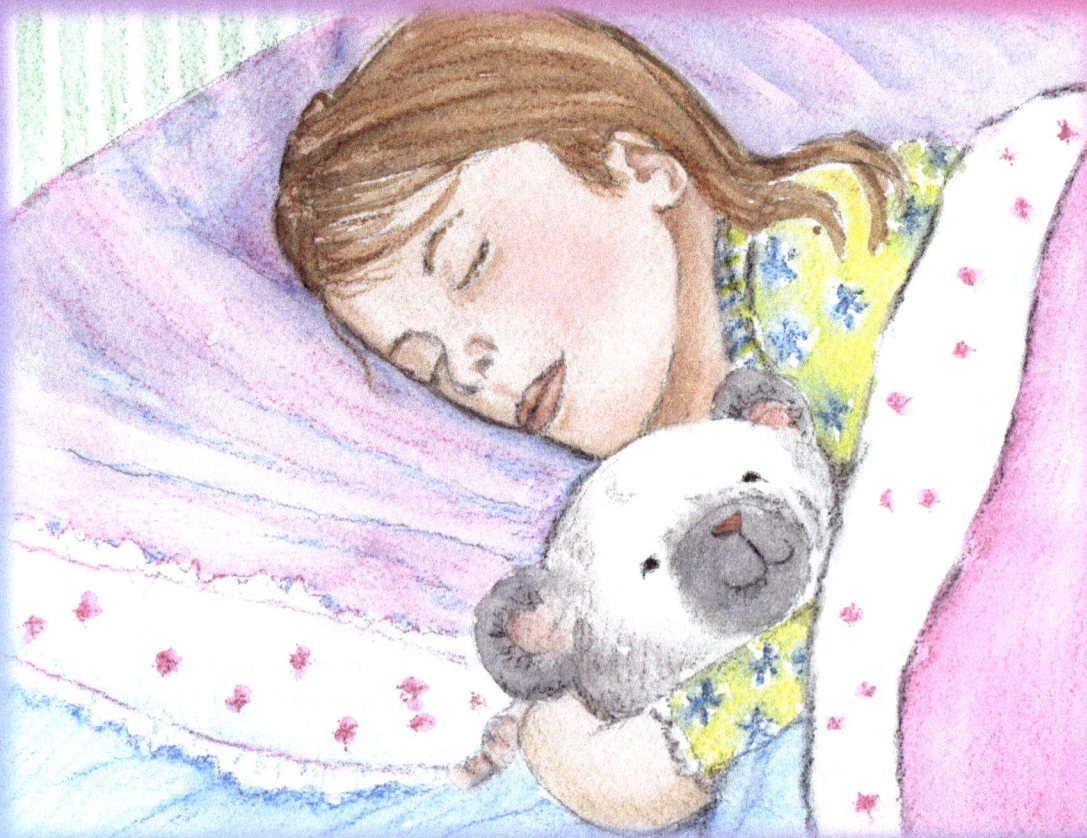

...or I can breathe on purpose.

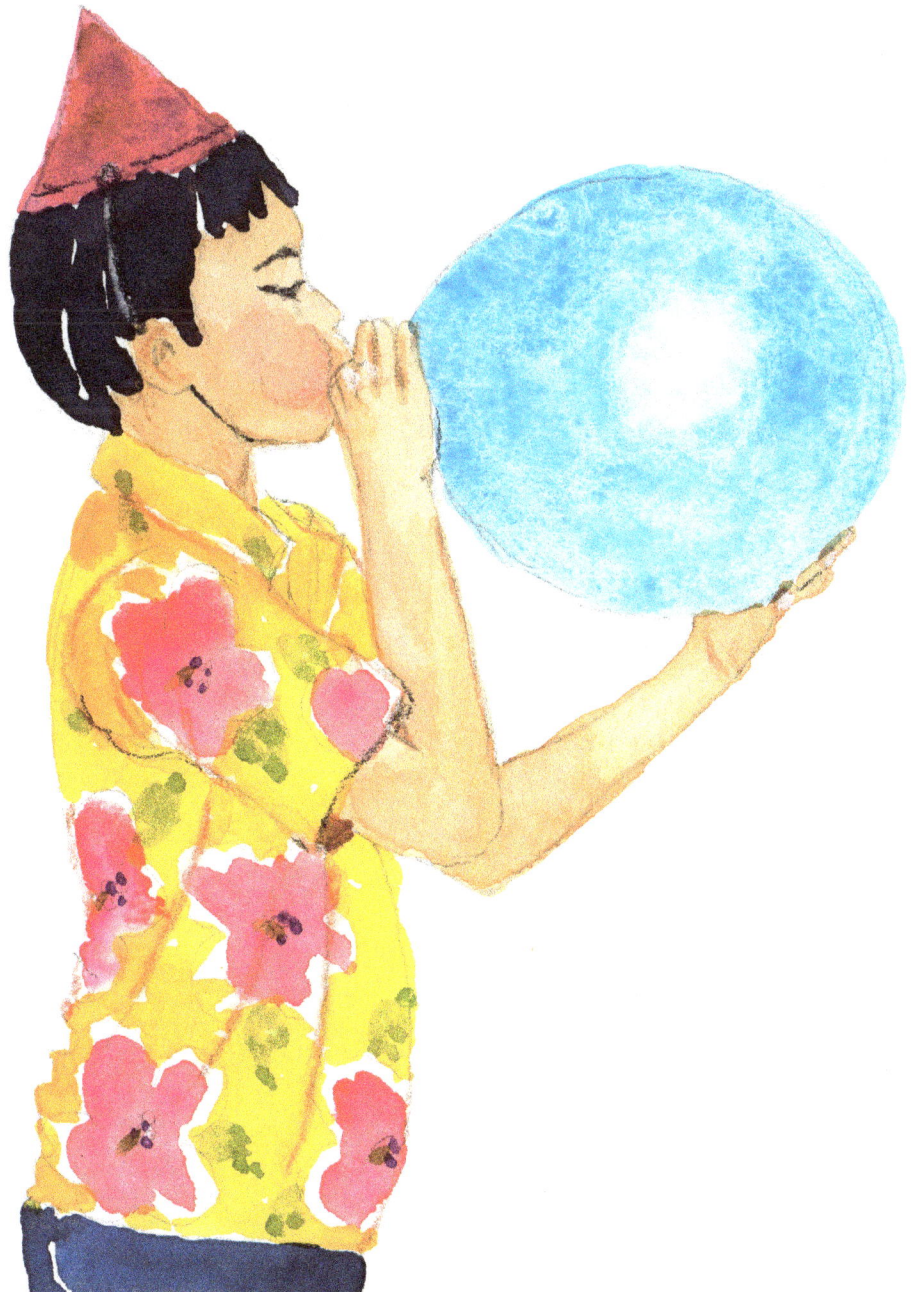

I can breathe through my nose,

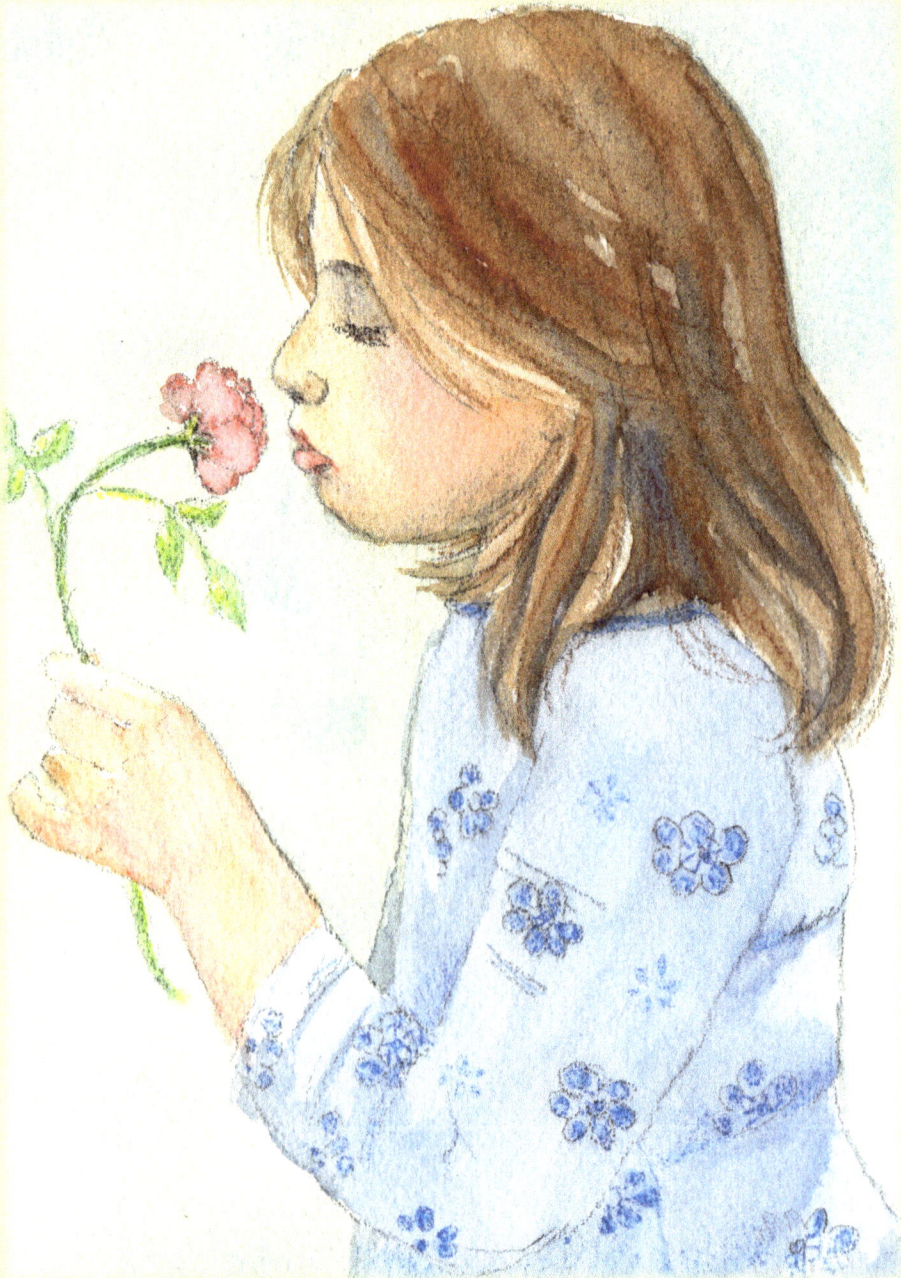

or through
my mouth,

or both.

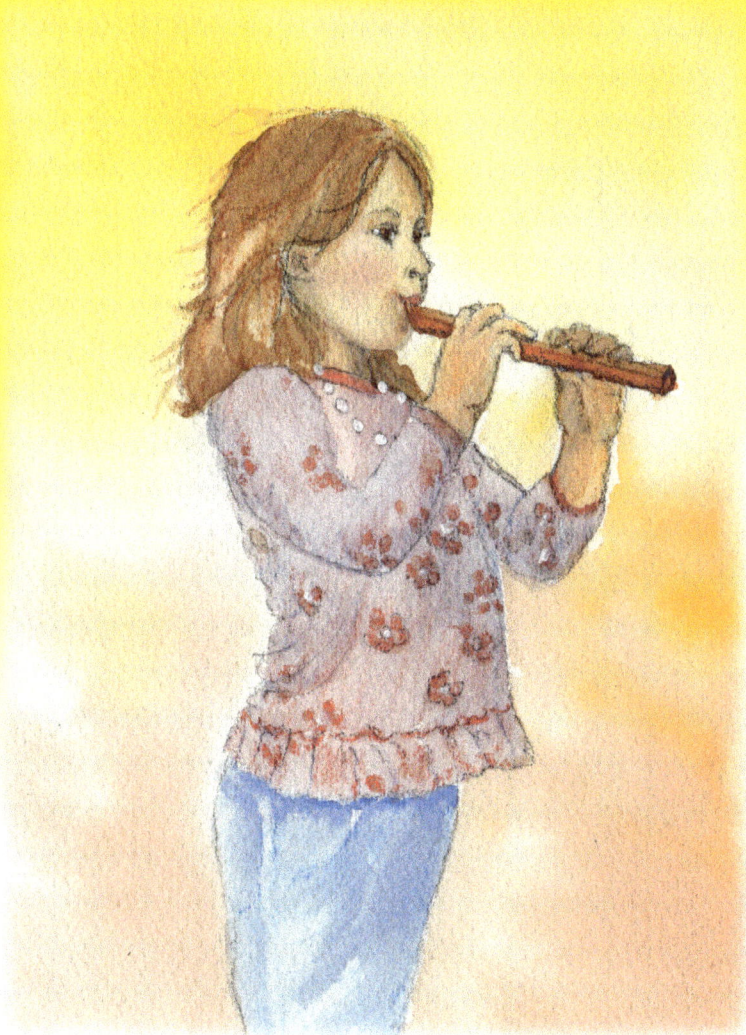

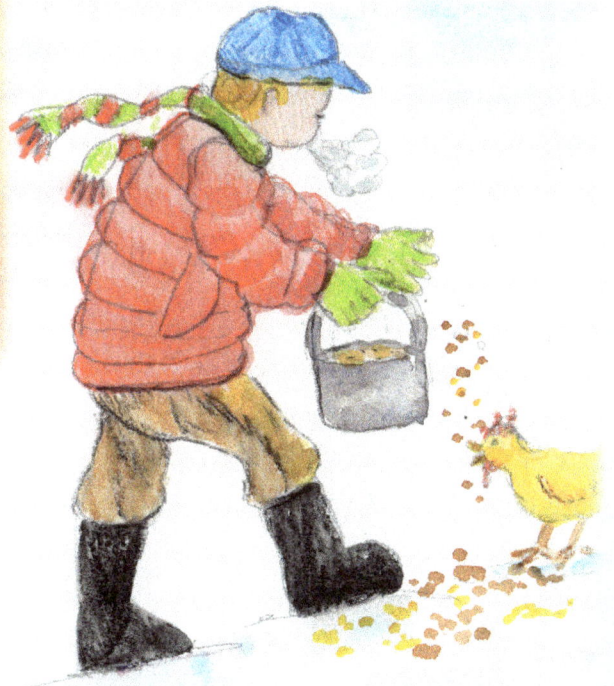

What does

my breath

sound like?

It sounds like

the wind.

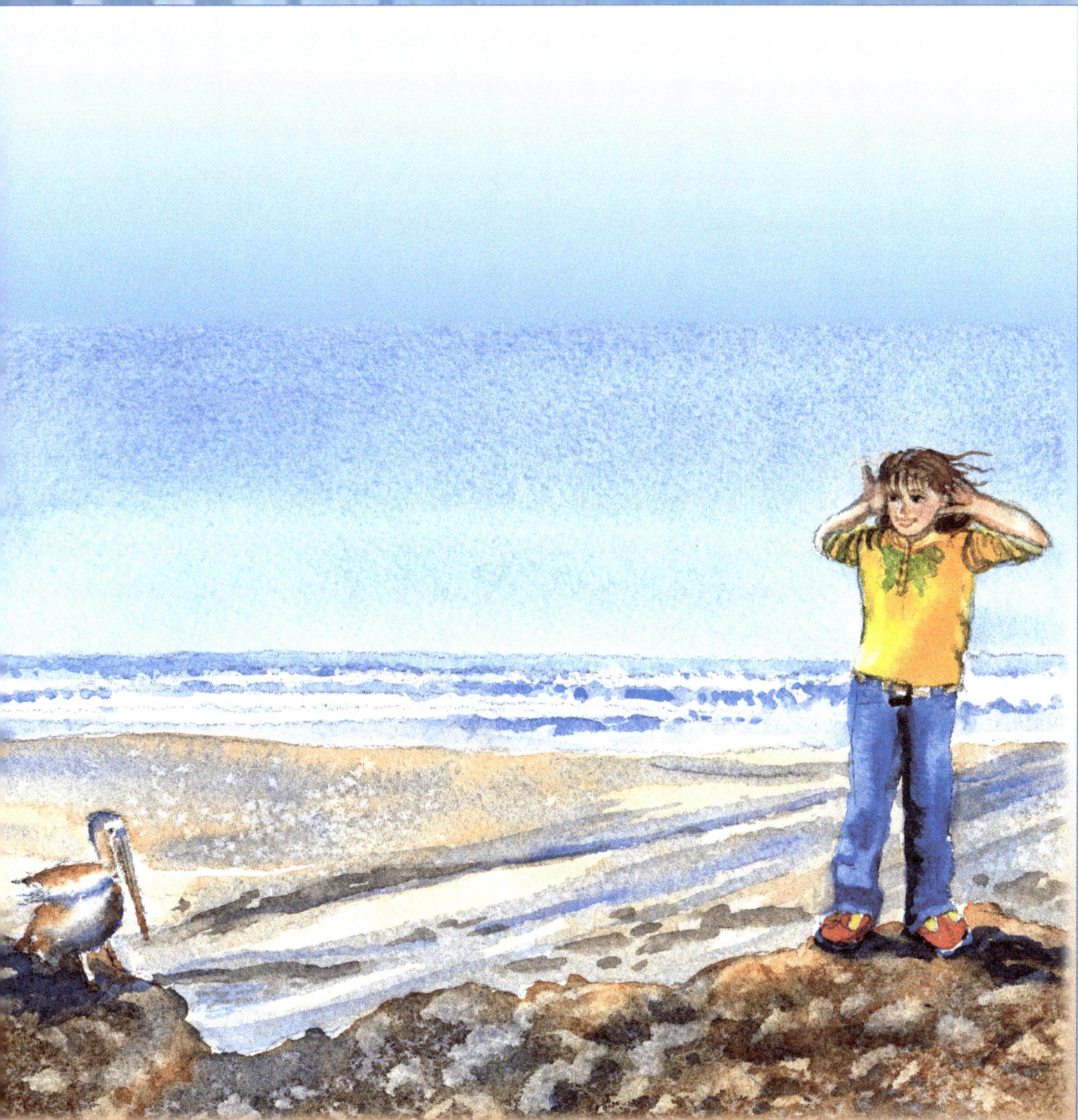

I breathe in the wind.

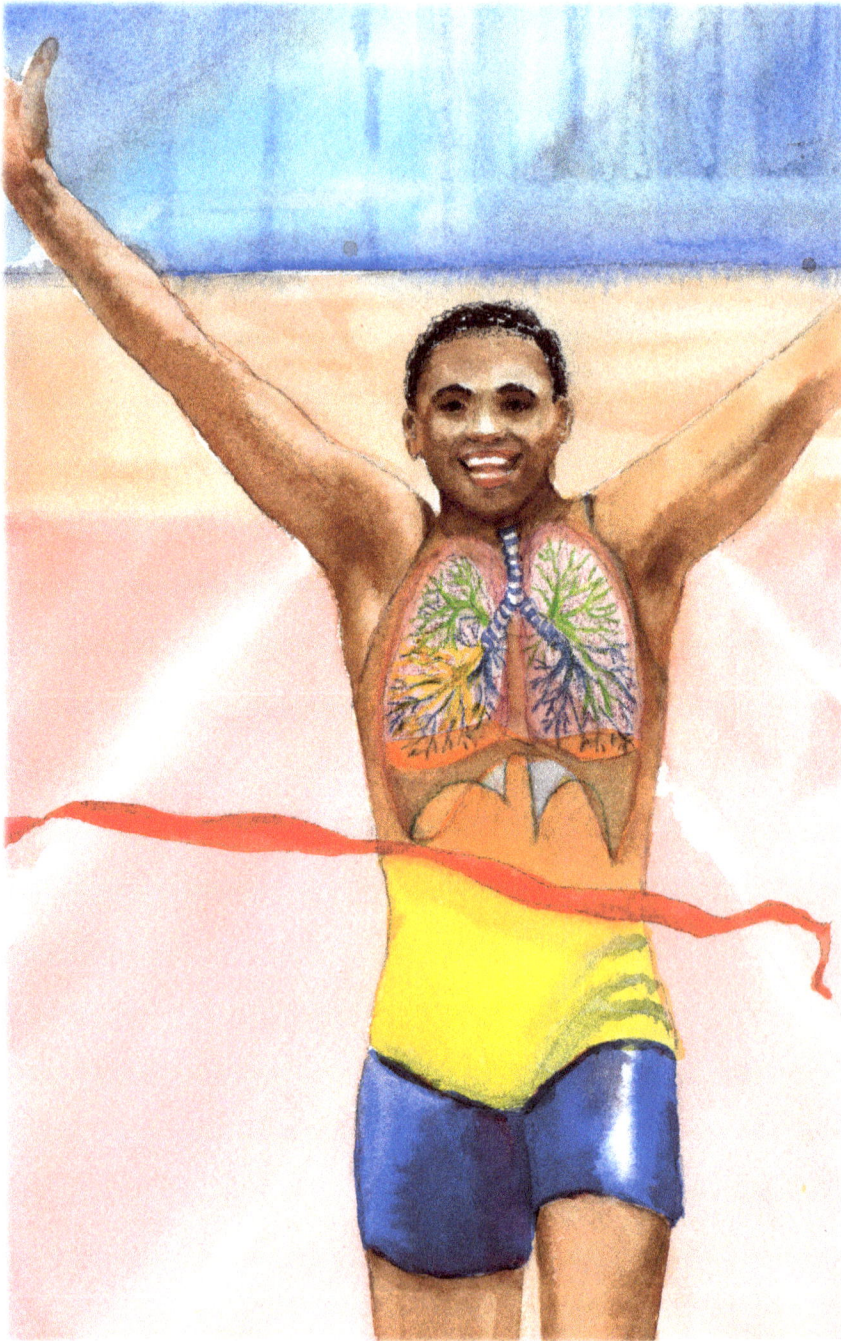

I inhale air into my lungs.

I can exhale the wind, too.

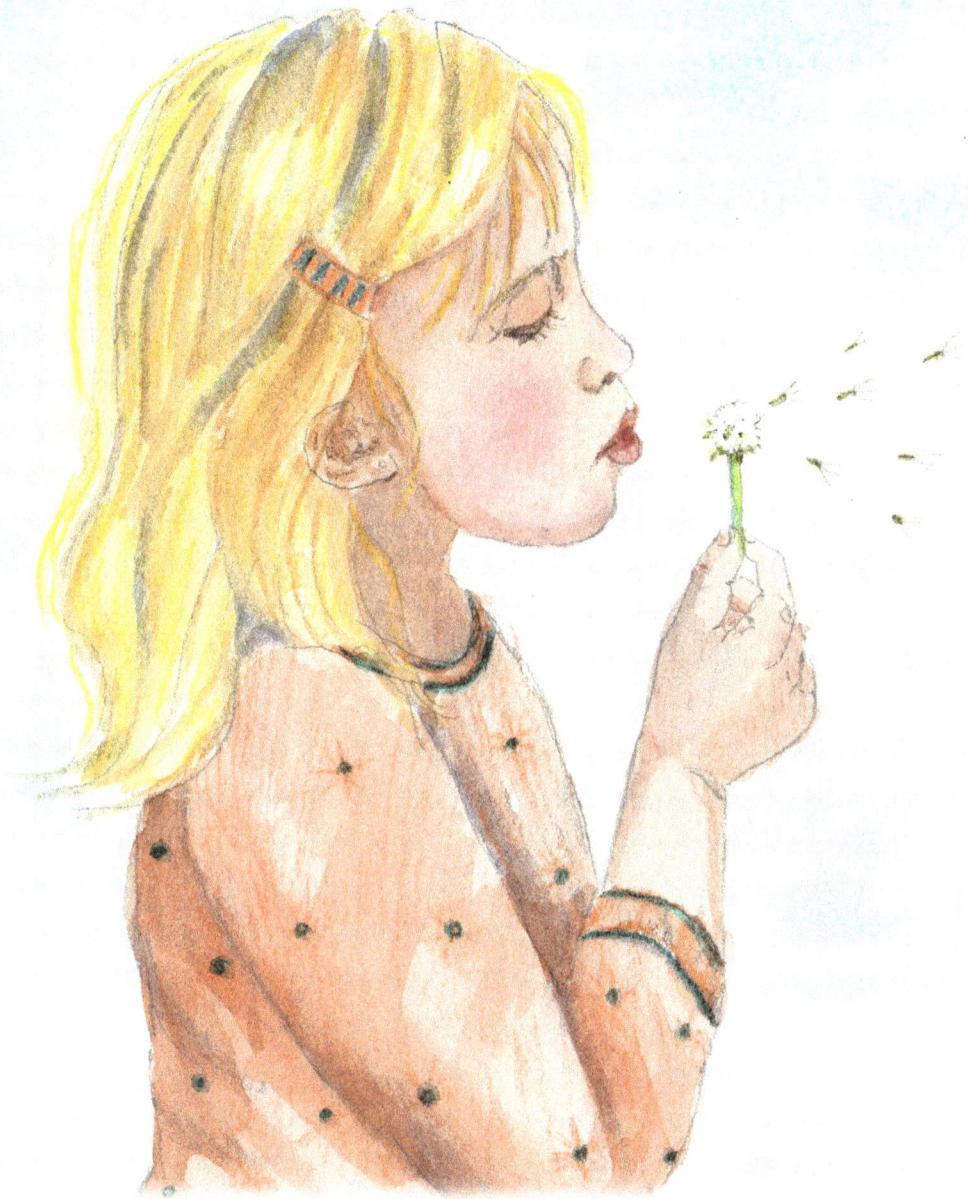

When I breathe out,
I have the power of the
Wind.

Exhaling gives me power to jump,

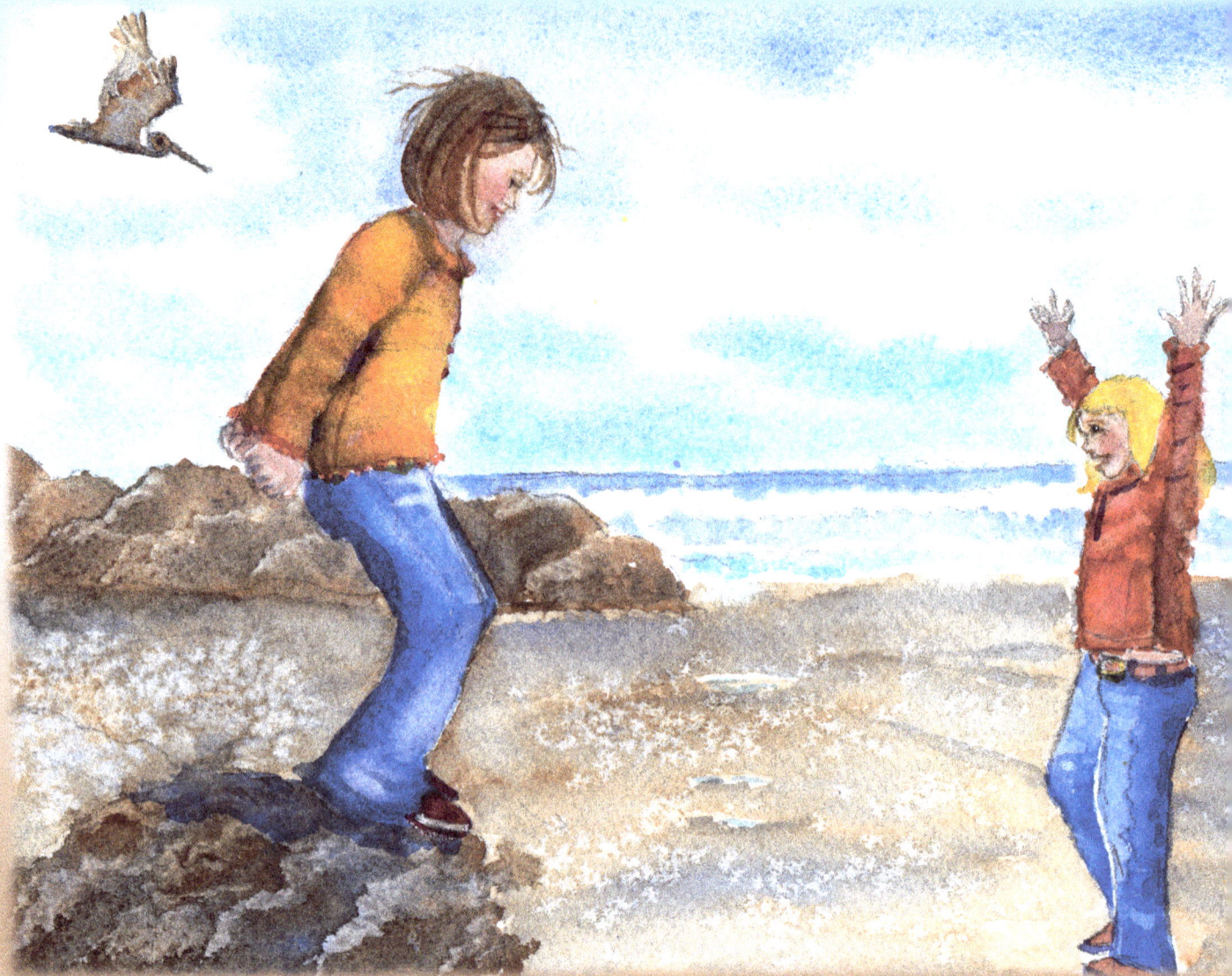

power to run,

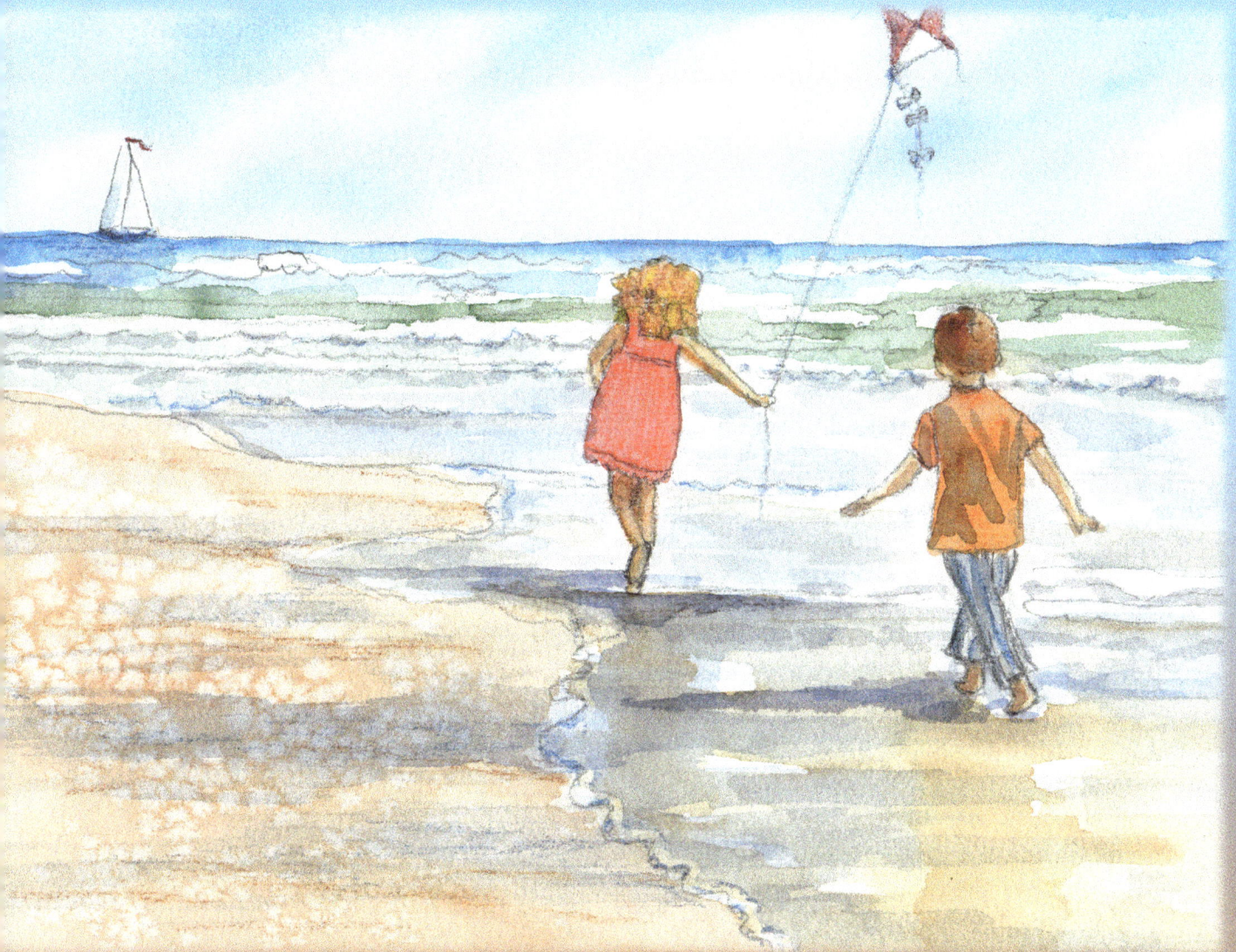

power to play and have fun!

We watch our bellies go
round as we inhale,

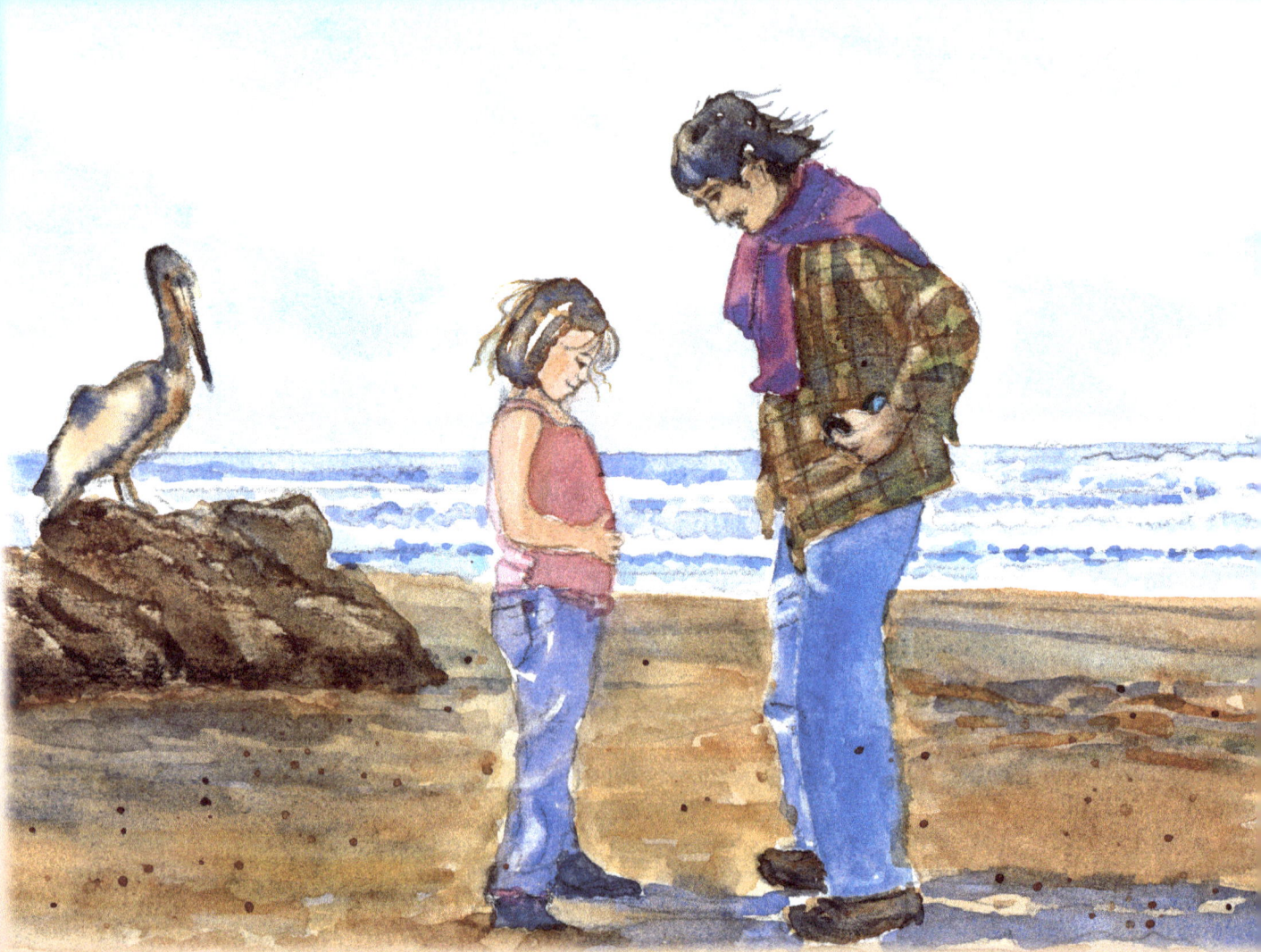

and flatten out as we exhale.

If I inhale as I turn the page...

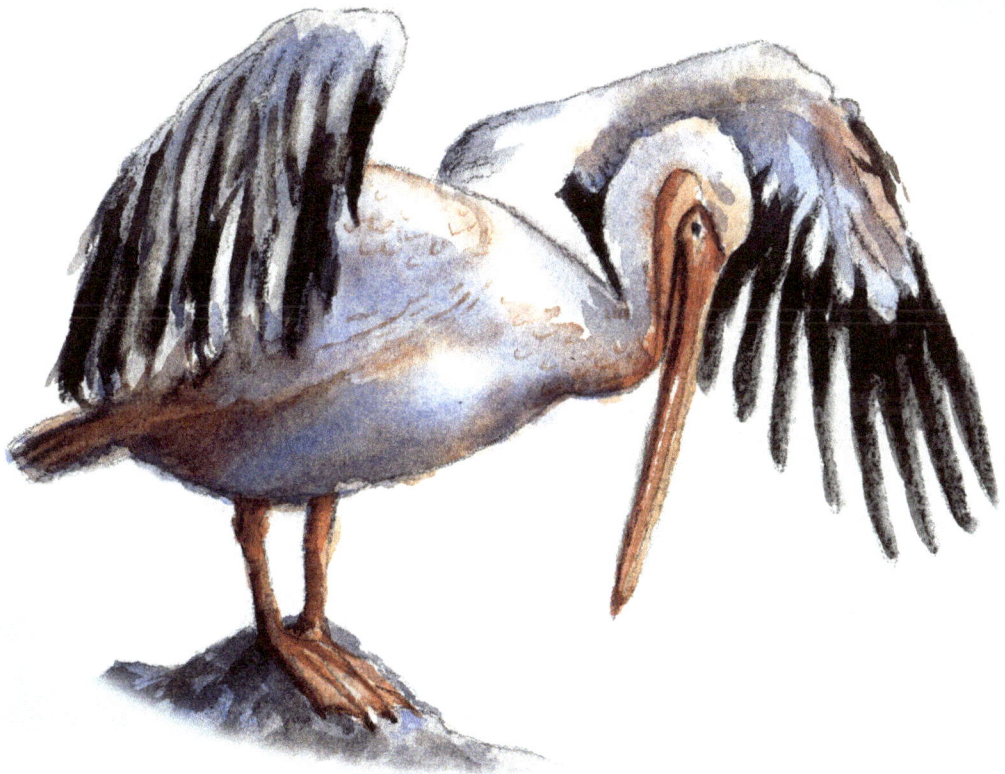

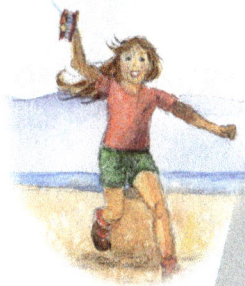

inhale

I will breathe out as
I read these
words out loud.

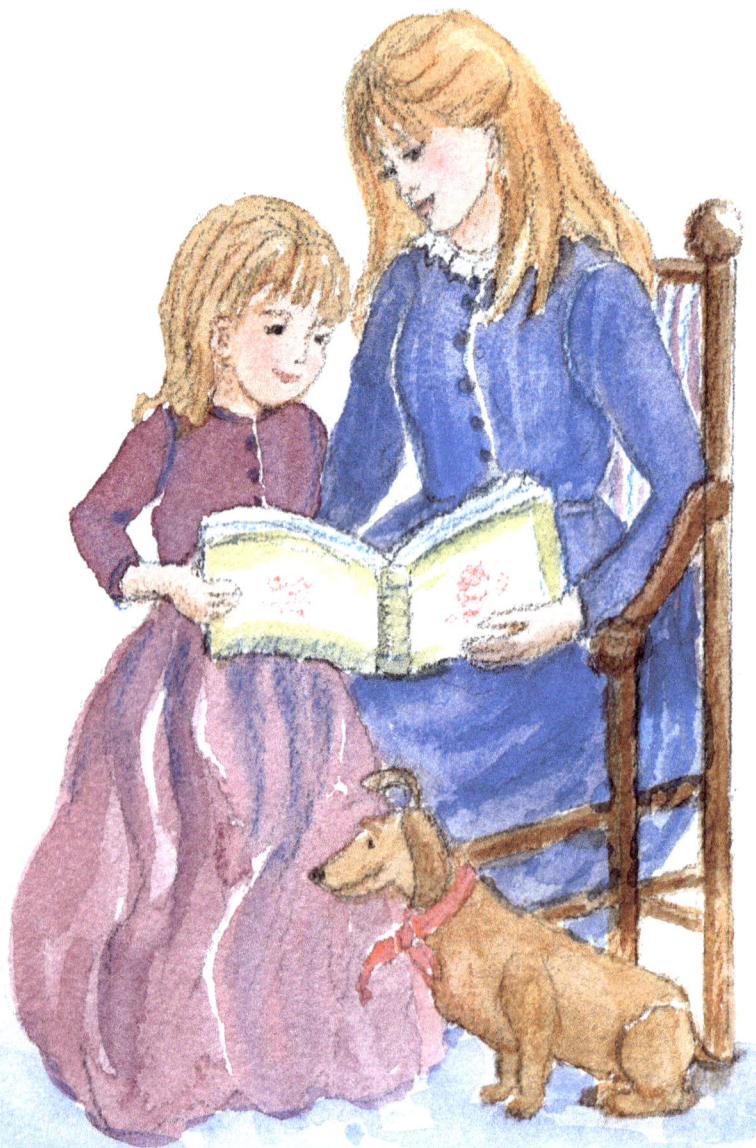

I breathe out when I say

"Hi" to my friend.

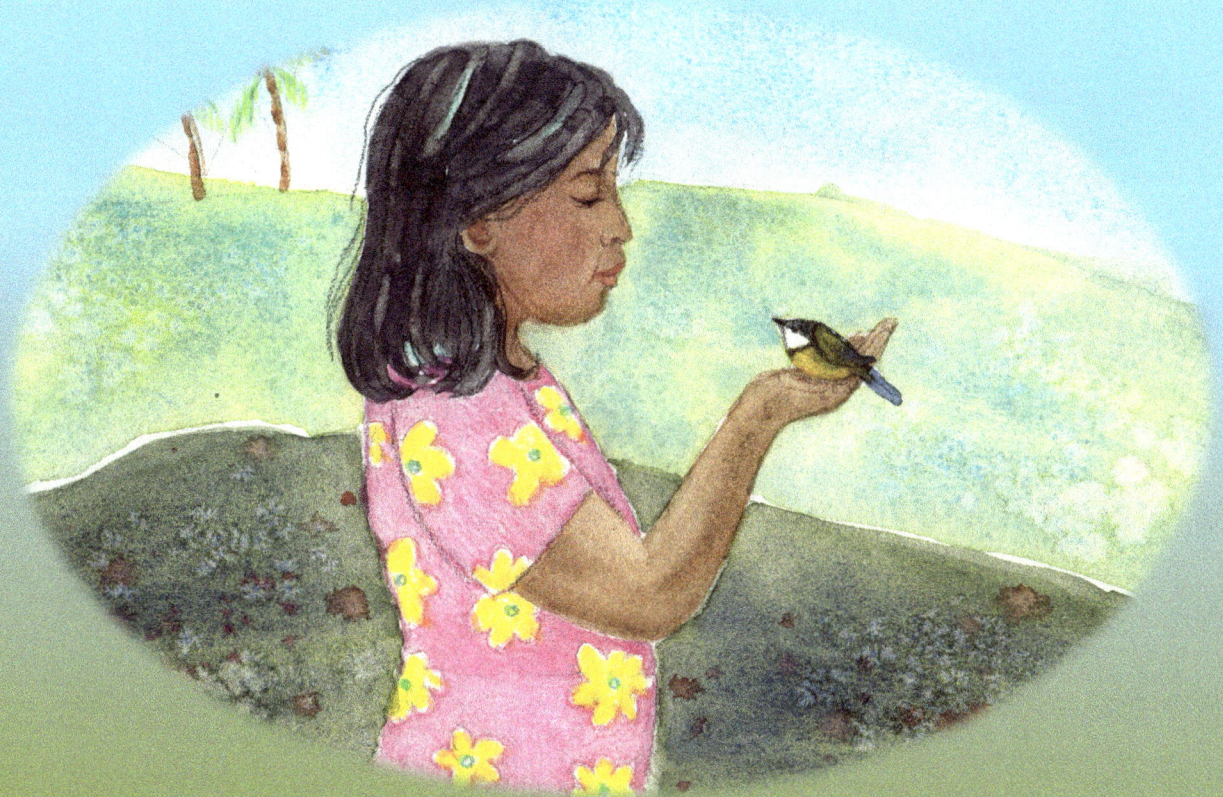

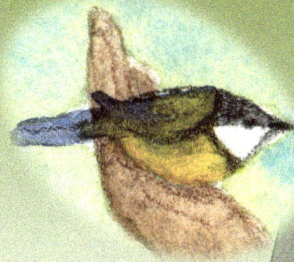

inhale

I exhale when I blow out candles,

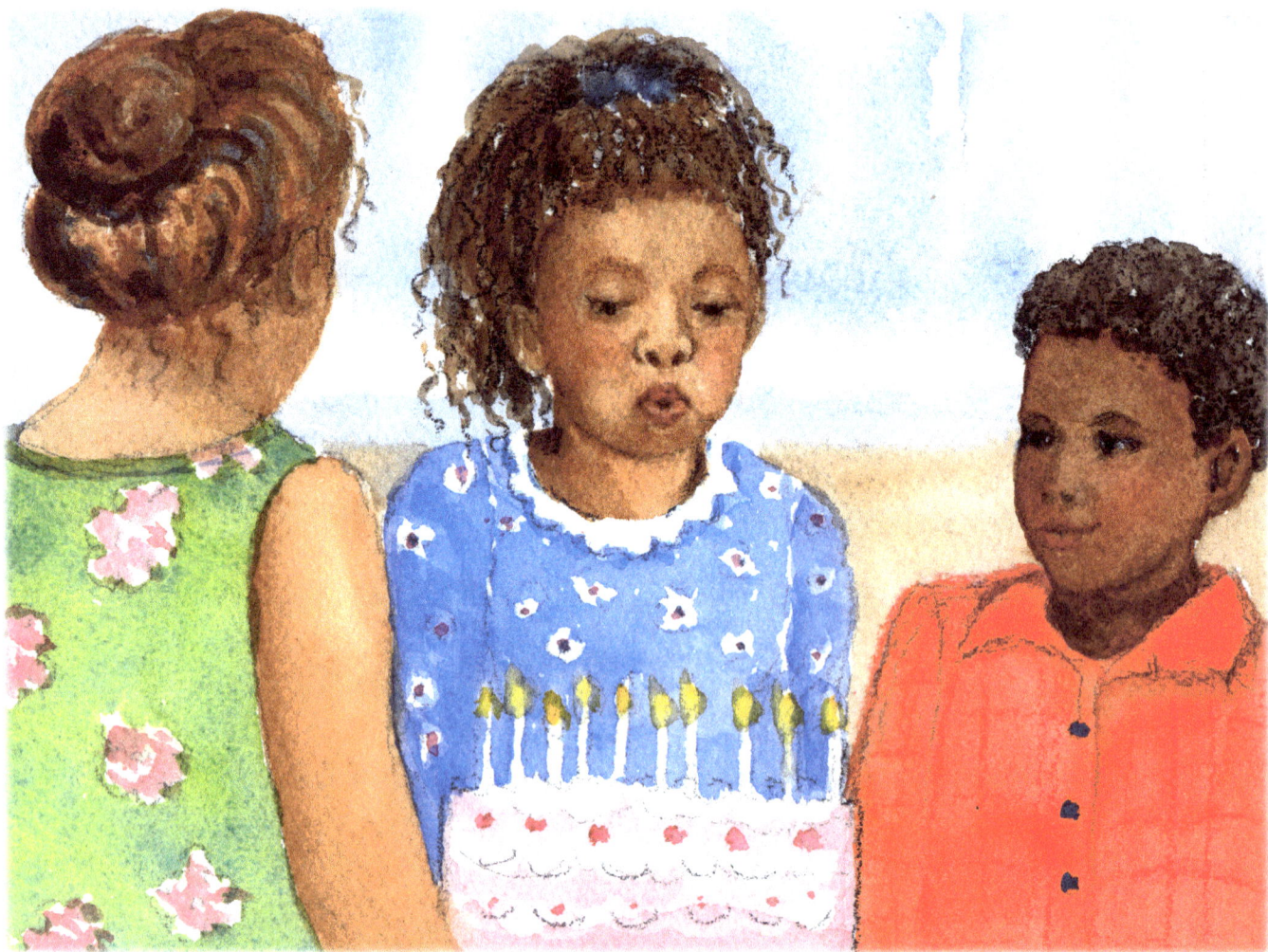

and when I laugh.

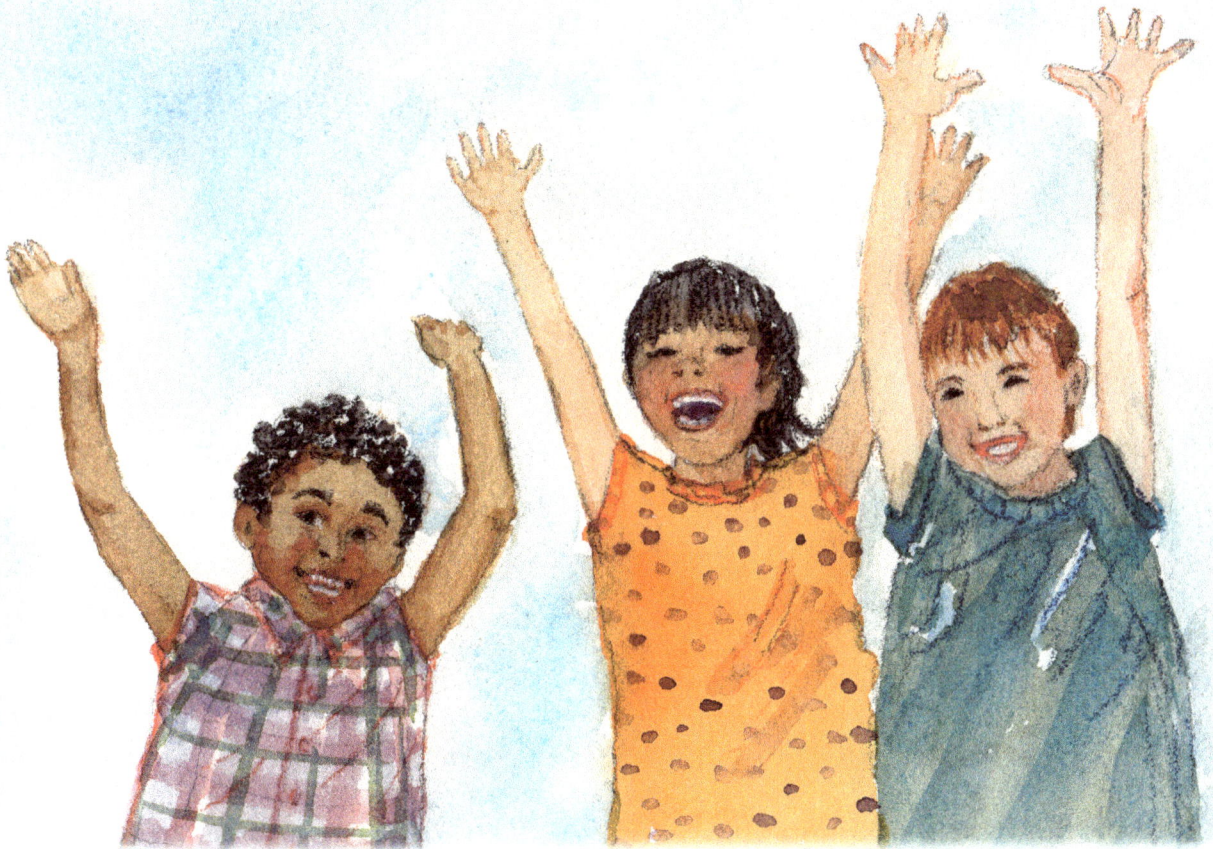

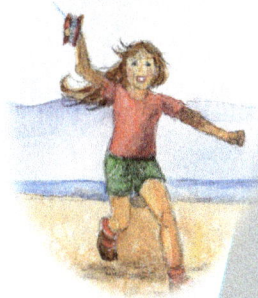

inhale

I breathe out when I
whisper a secret,

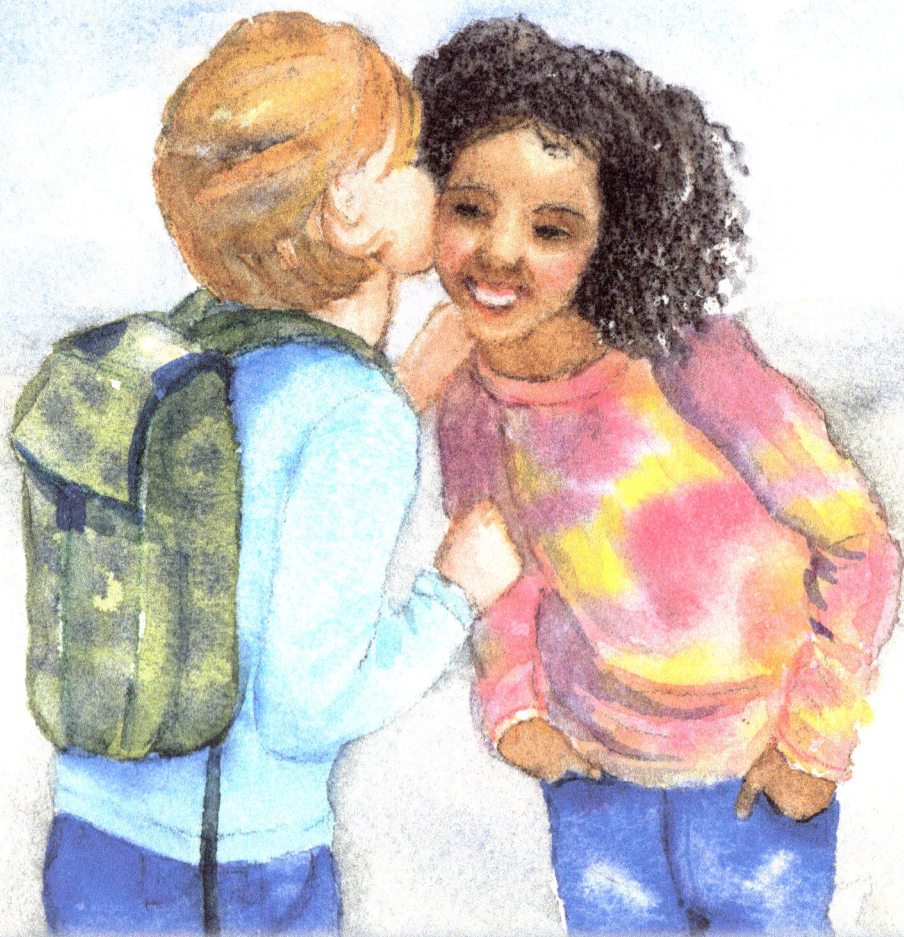

and when I sigh –

a sigh is a long exhale.

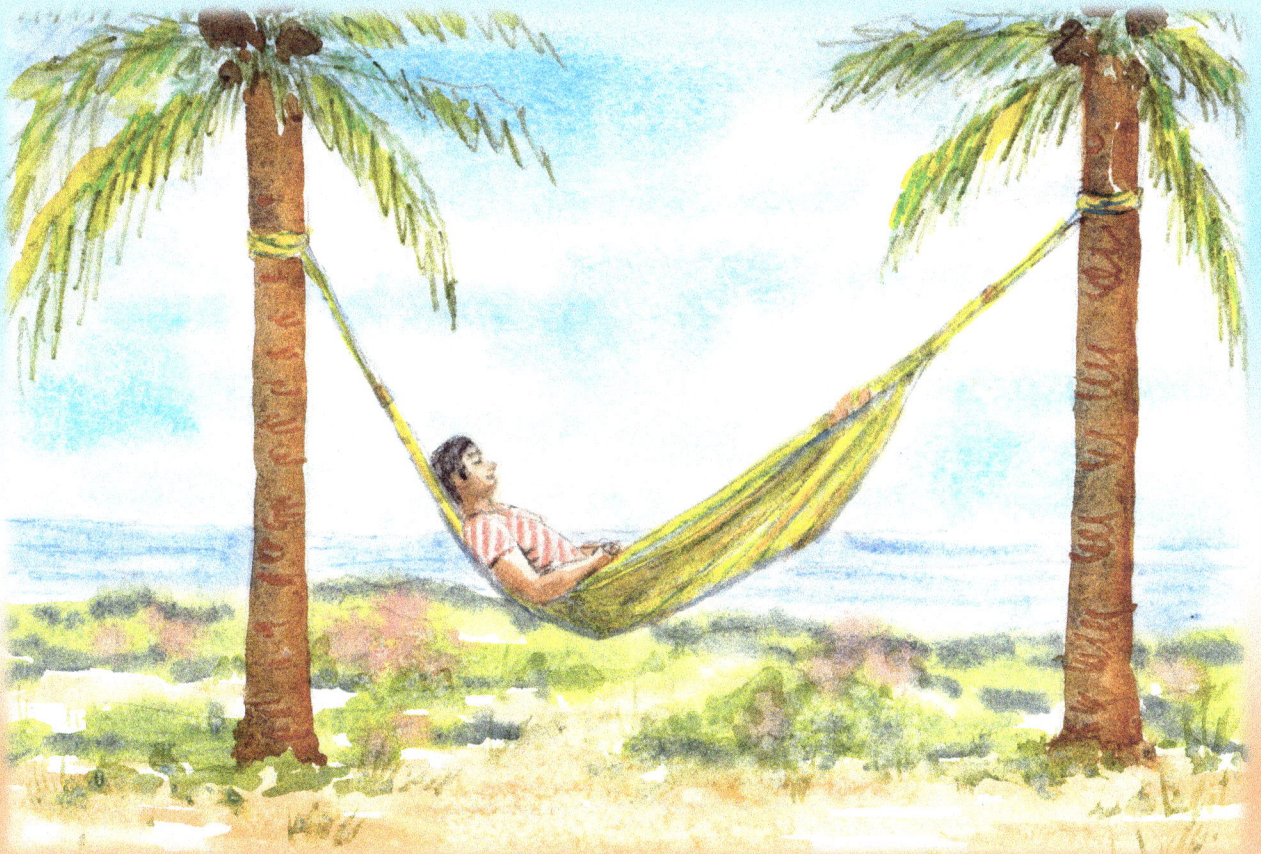

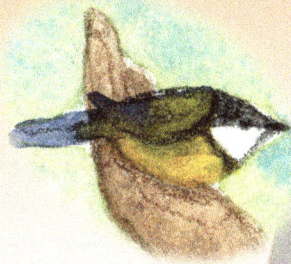

inhale

I exhale when I count to four,

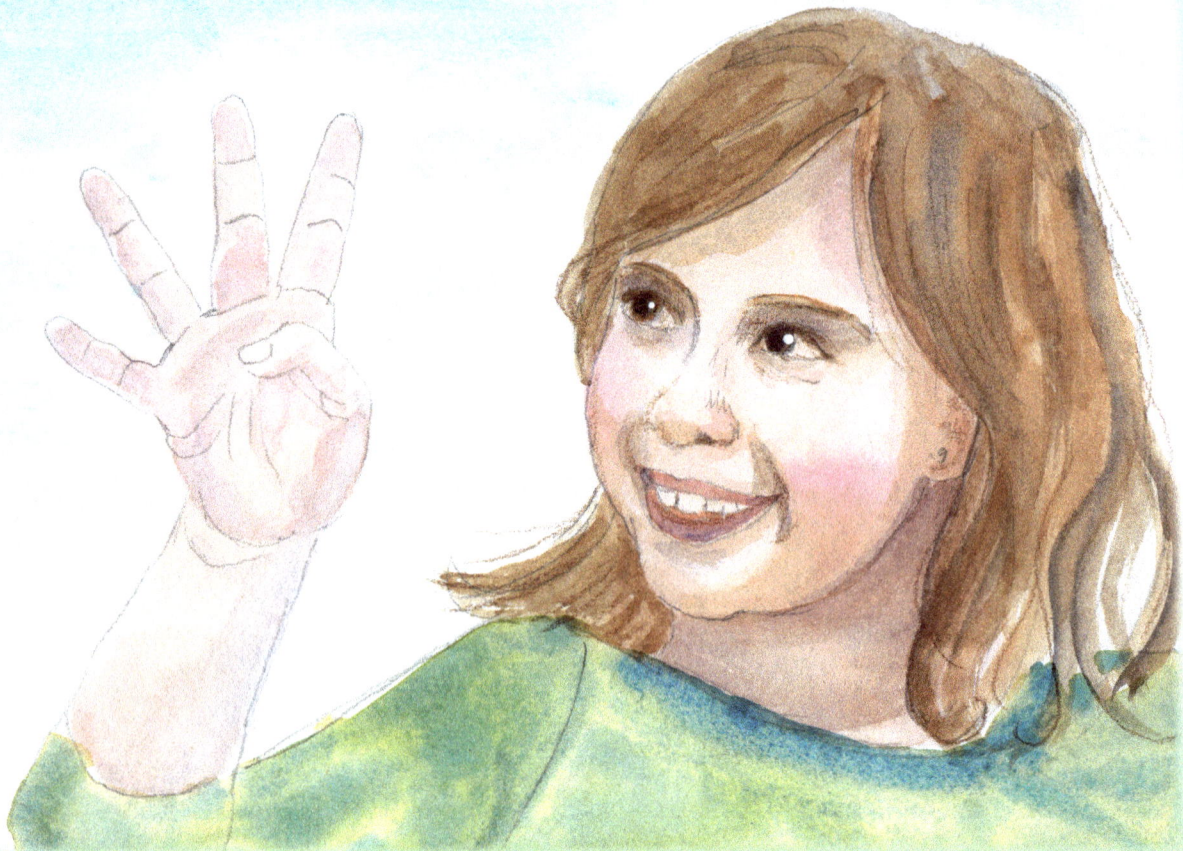

and when I do a chore.

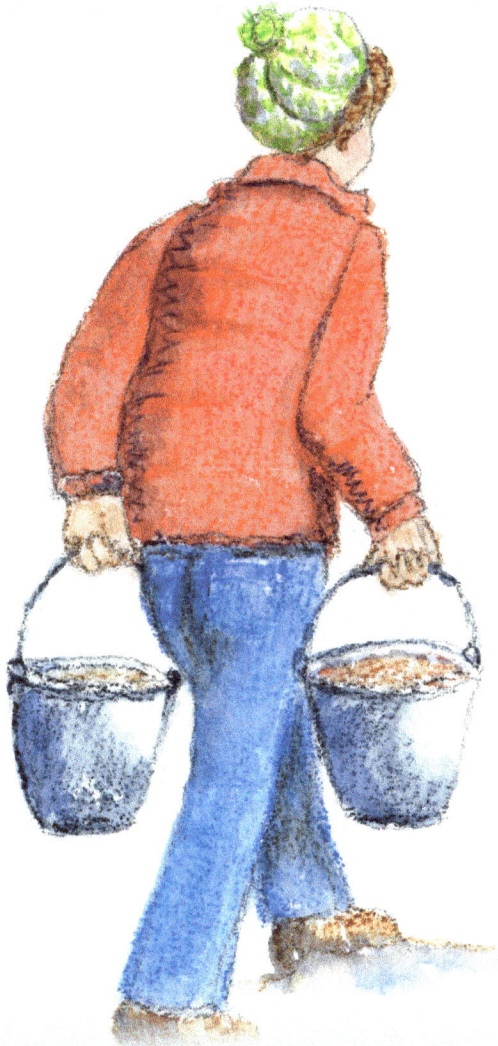

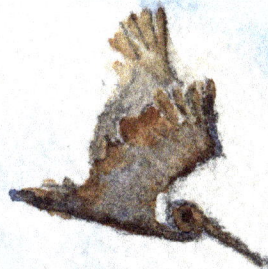

inhale

I breathe out when I whistle,

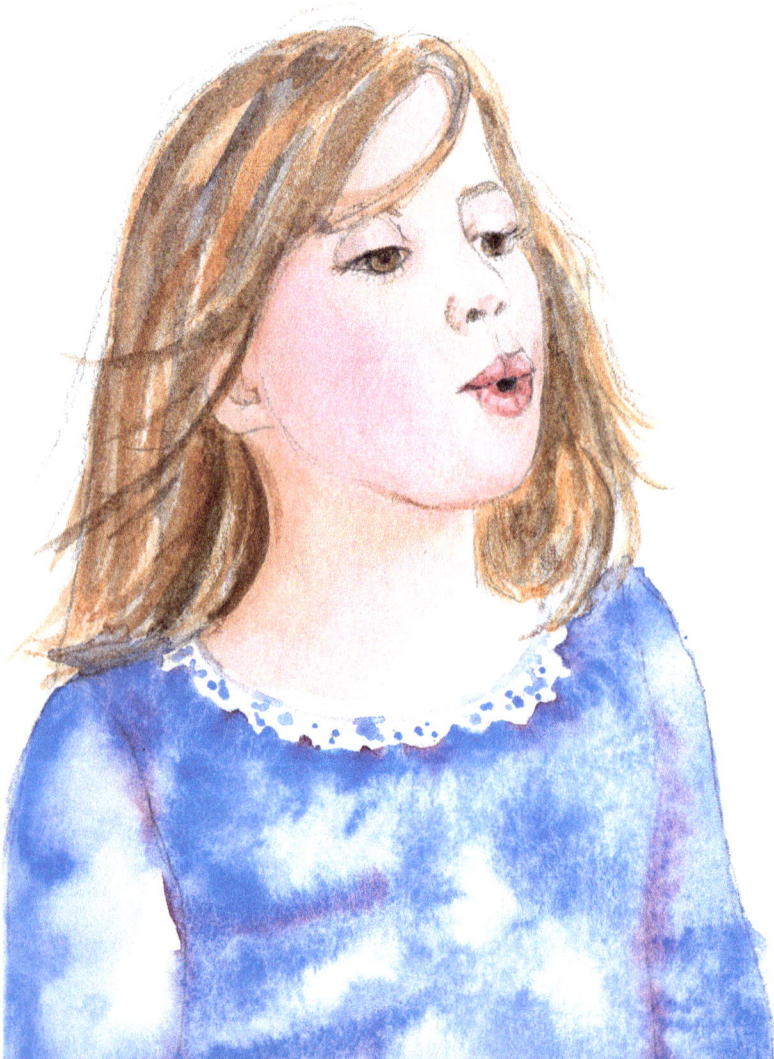

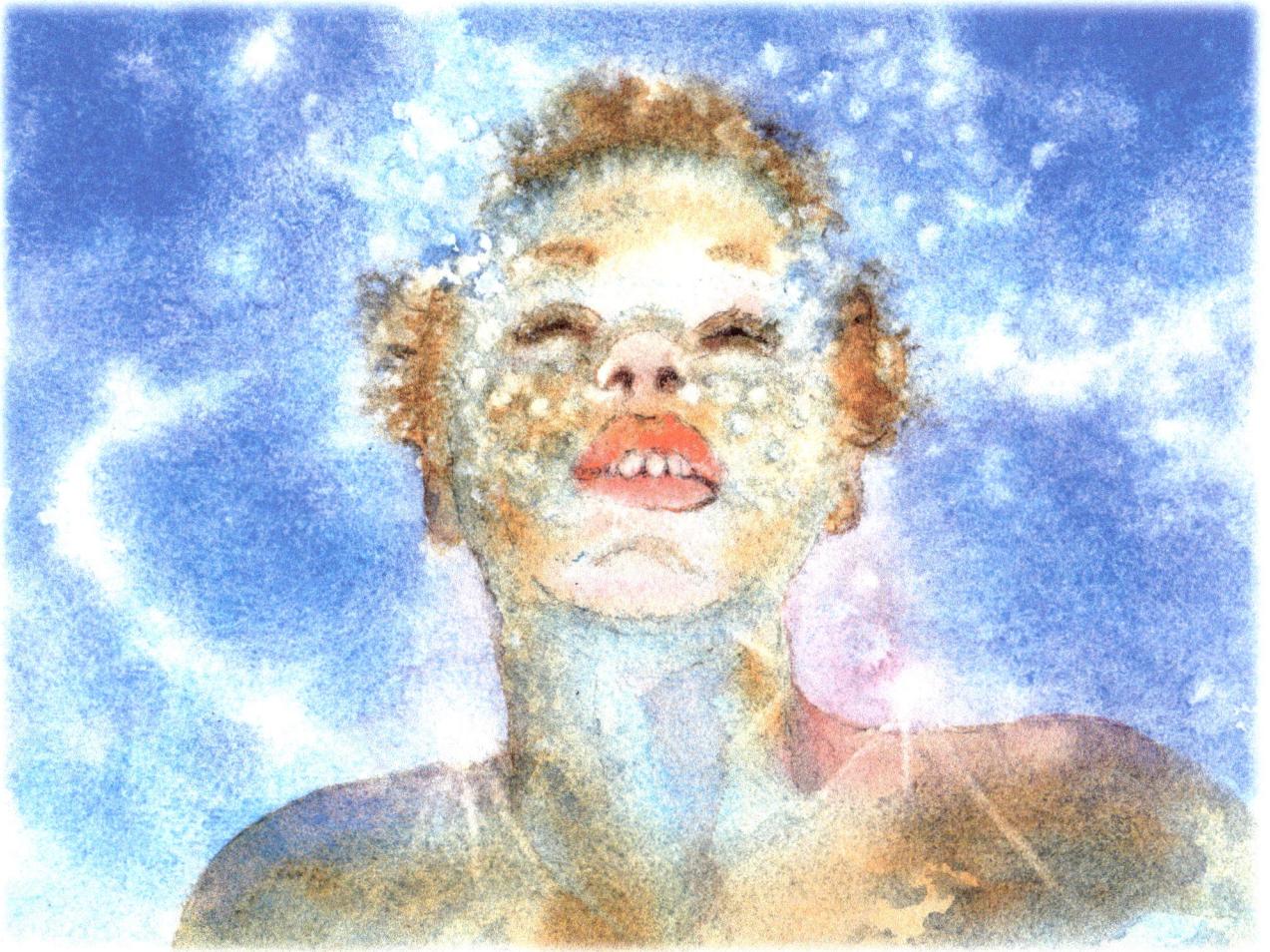

and when I swim under water –
even when I whistle under water!

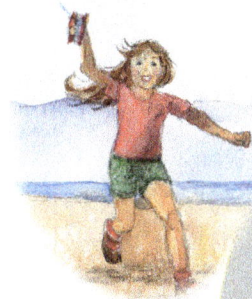

inhale

I exhale when I sing,

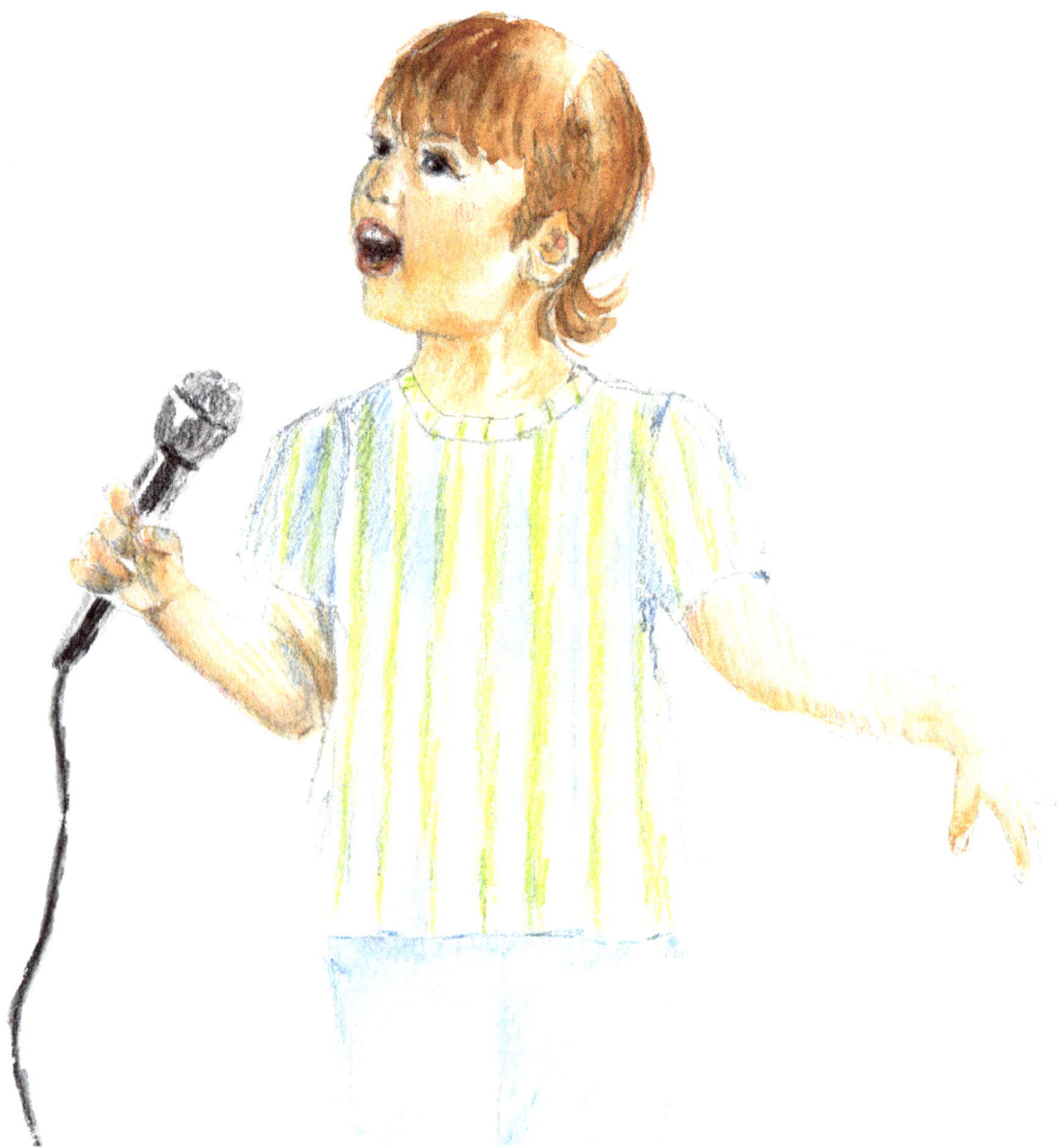

and when I dance.

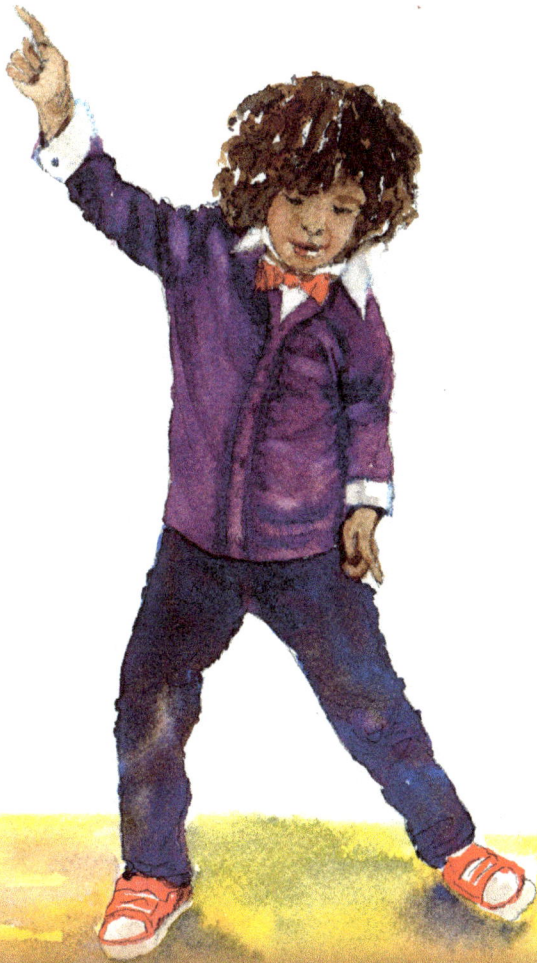

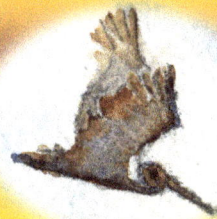

inhale

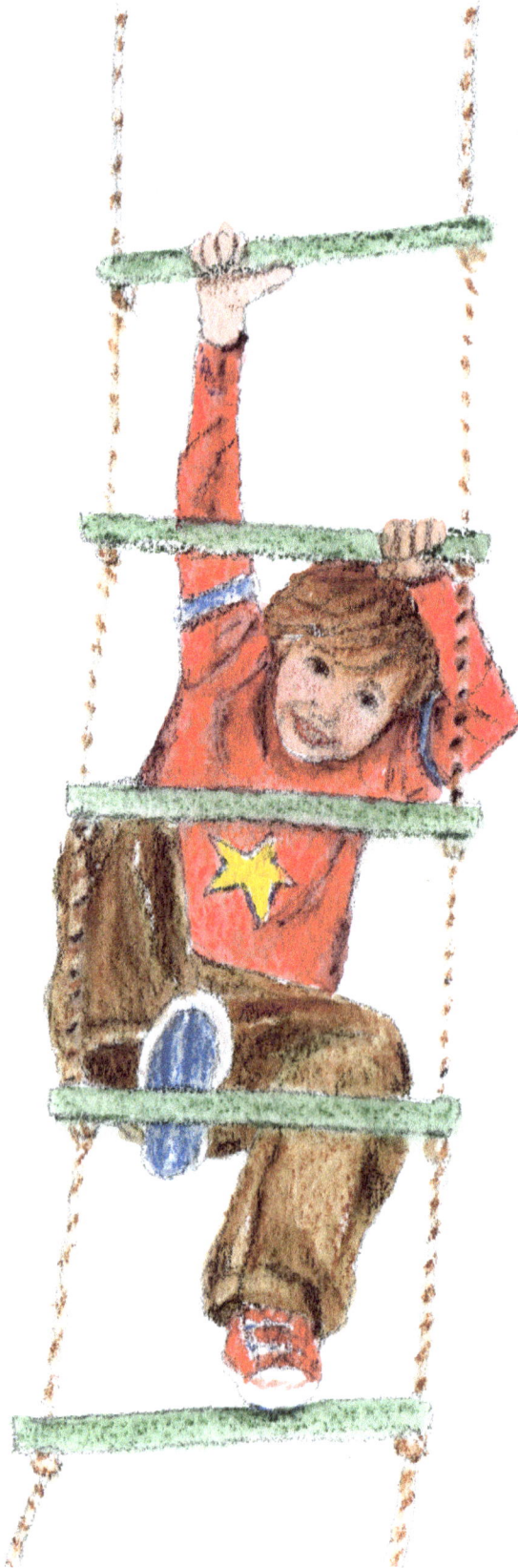

If I

breathe

out

when I

climb up

the ladder,

it's easier.

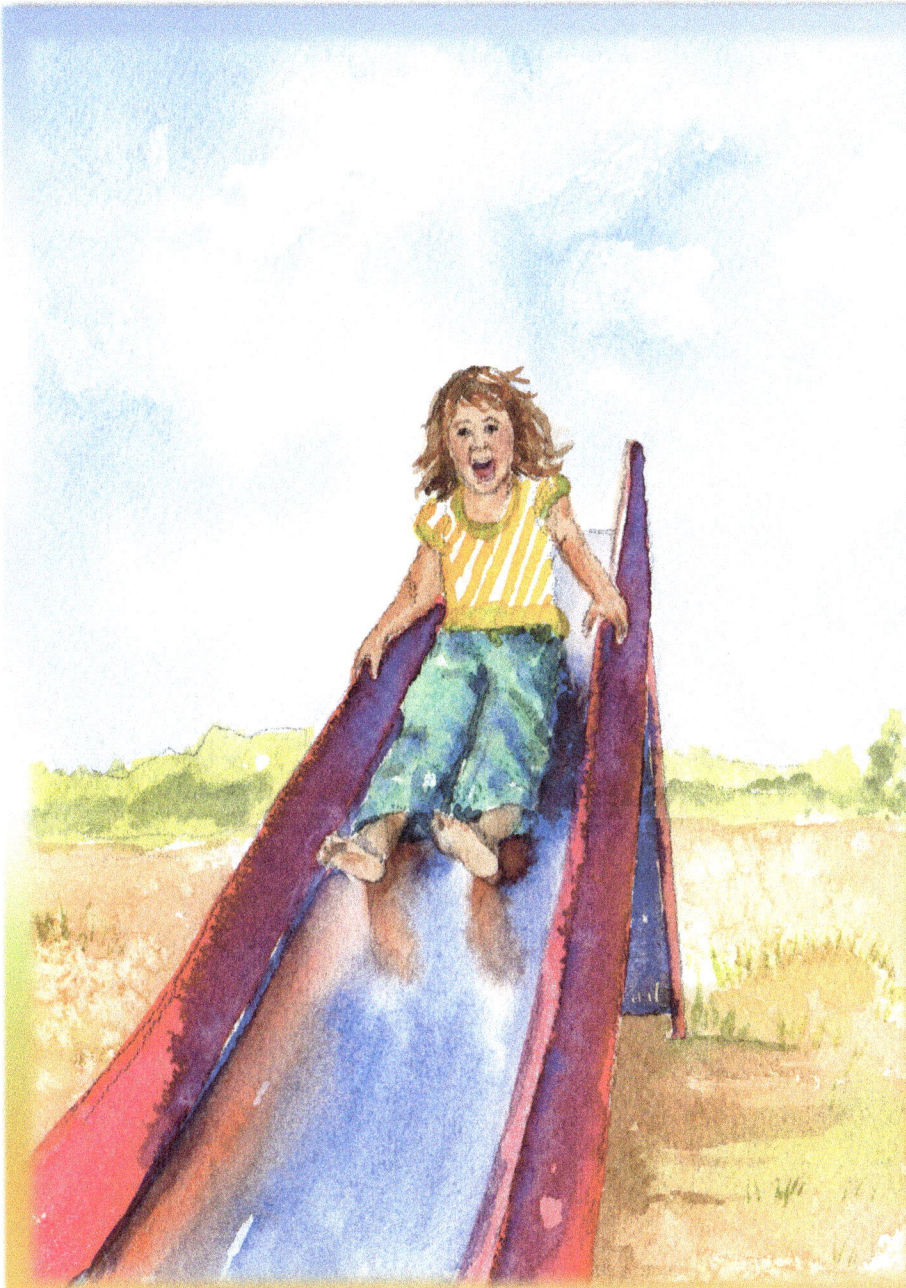

If I
breathe
out
when I
go down
the slide,
it's more
fun!

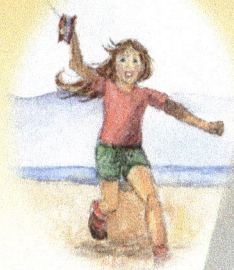

inhale

I exhale after I brush my teeth,

pah-tooey!

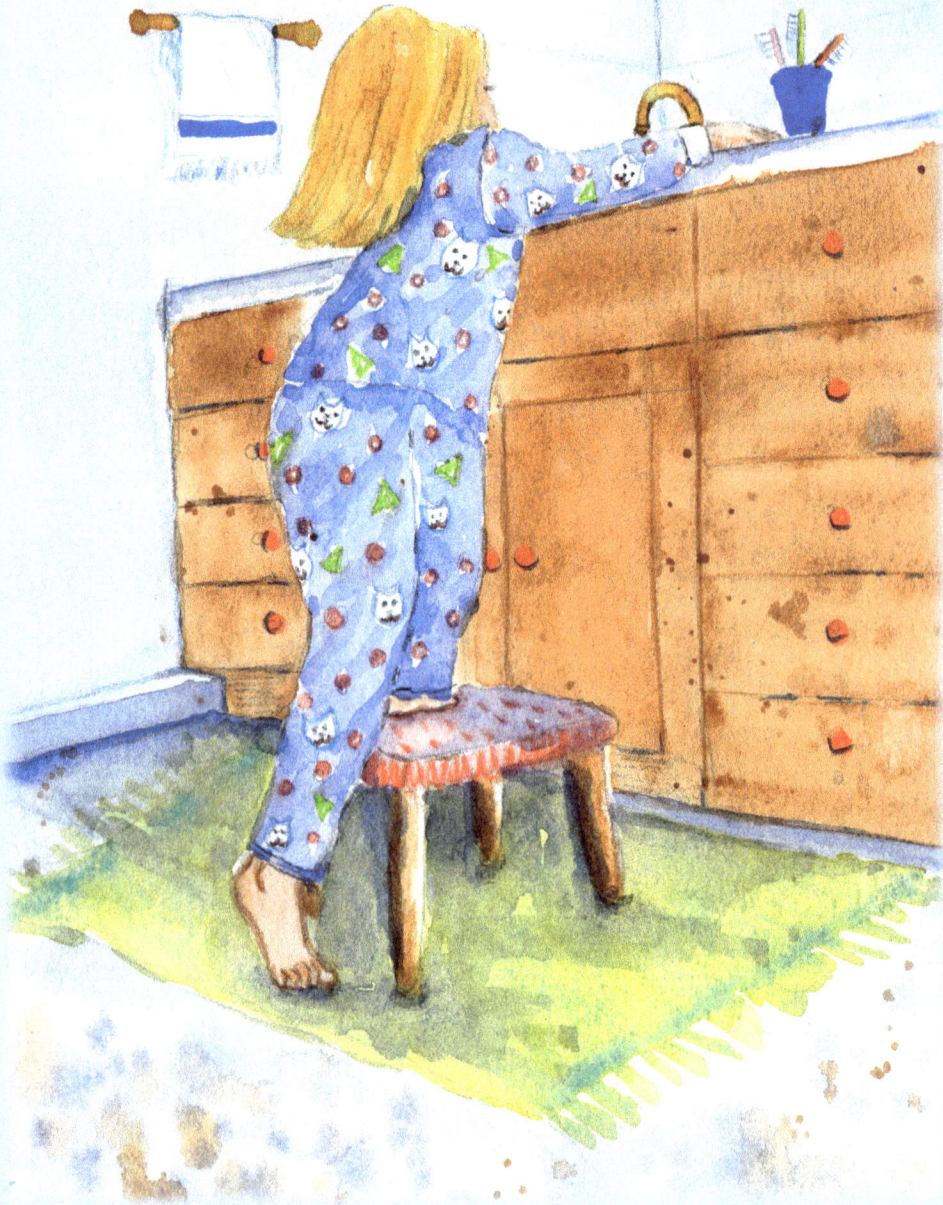

and when
I say,
"Good night."

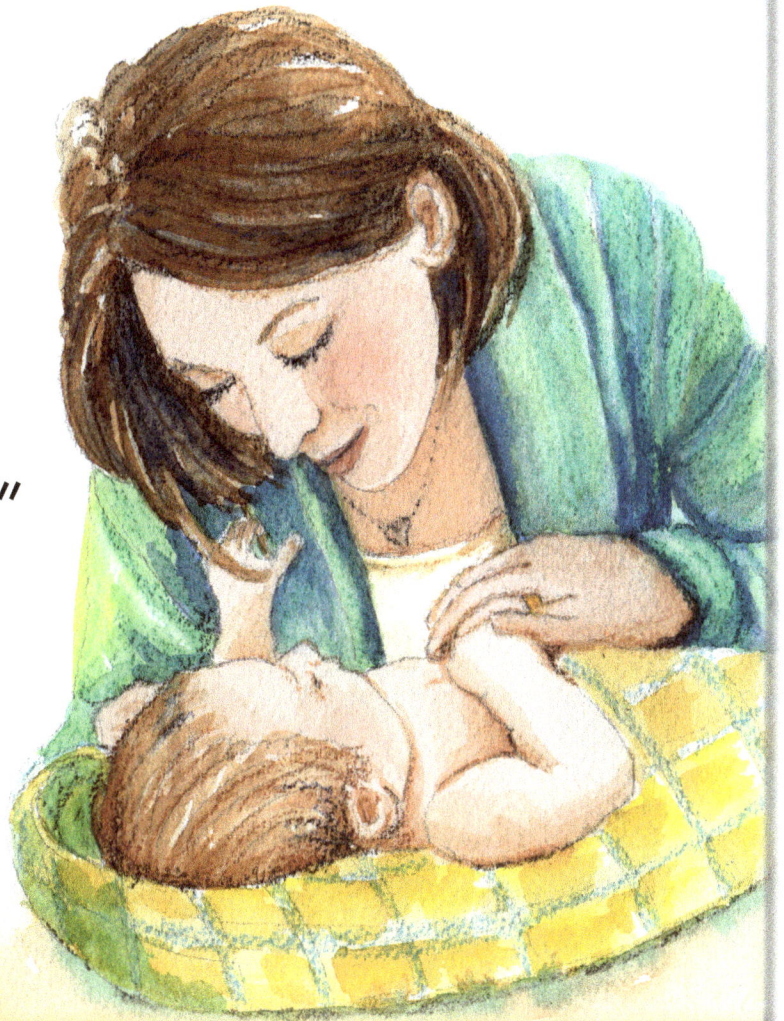

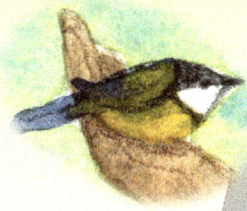

inhale

I breathe out when I say,

"Thank you,"

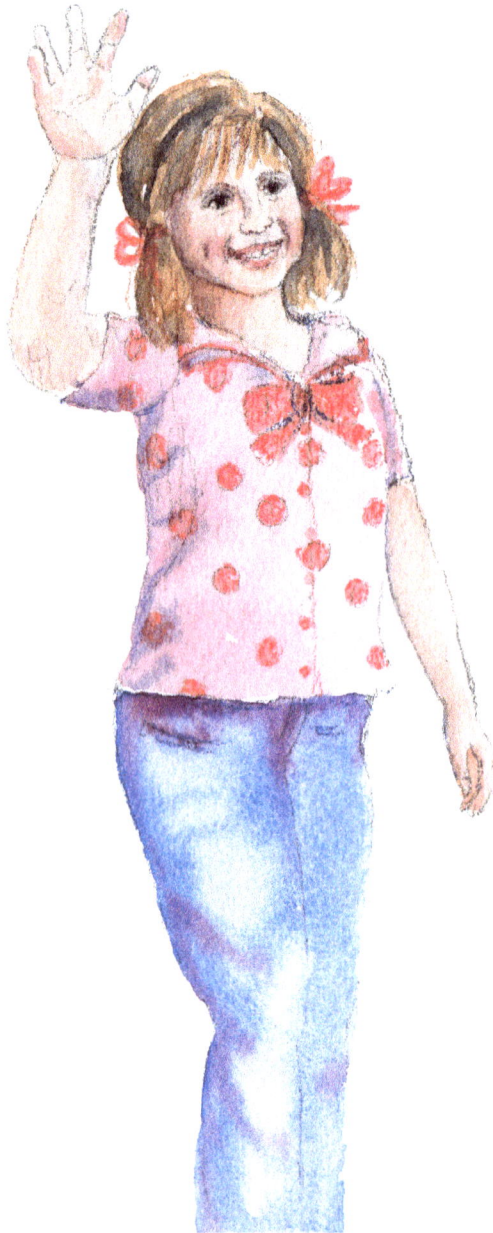

and when I say, "I love you."

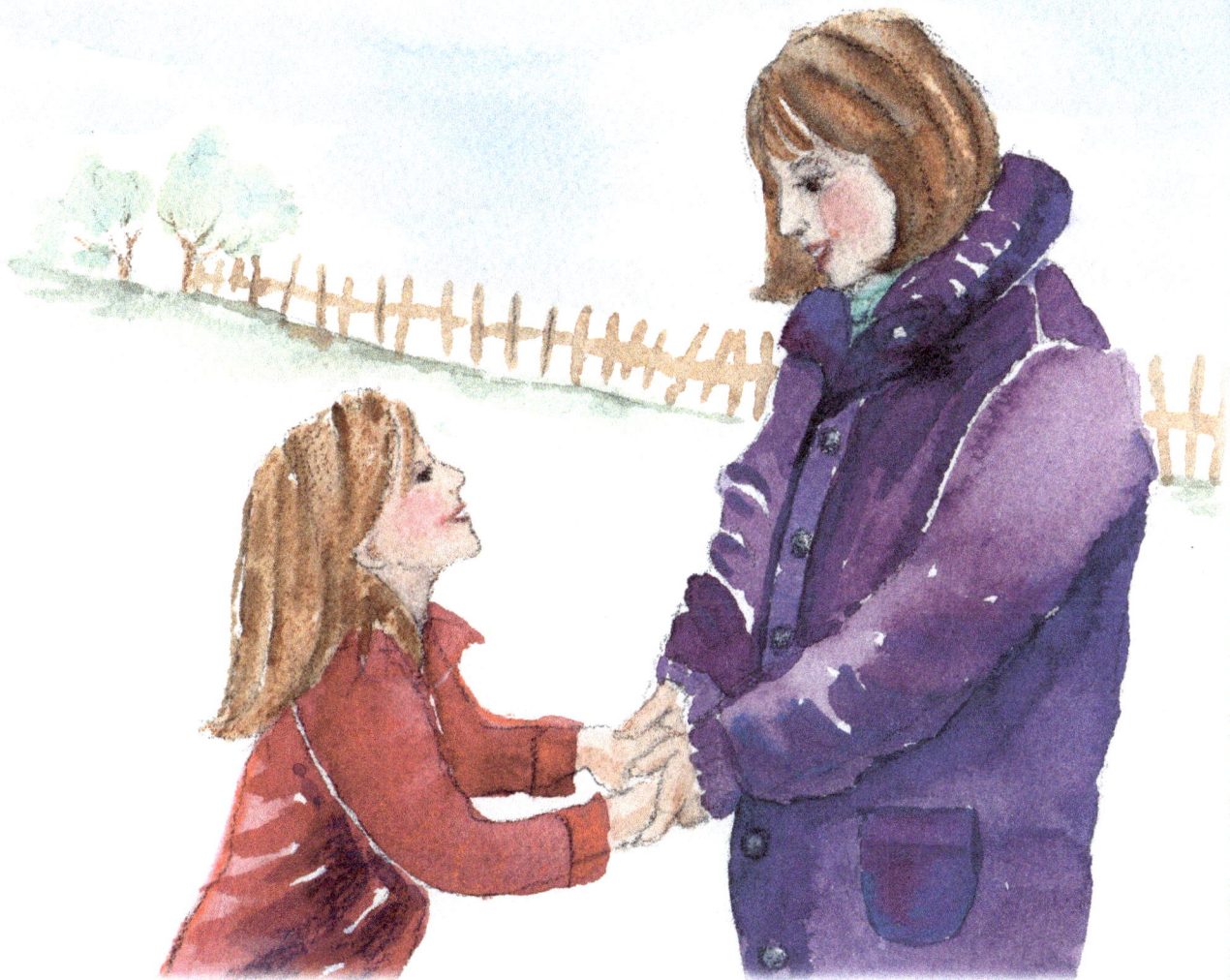

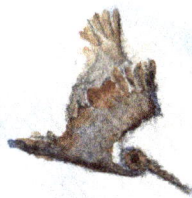

inhale

After all this exhaling,

I feel peace.

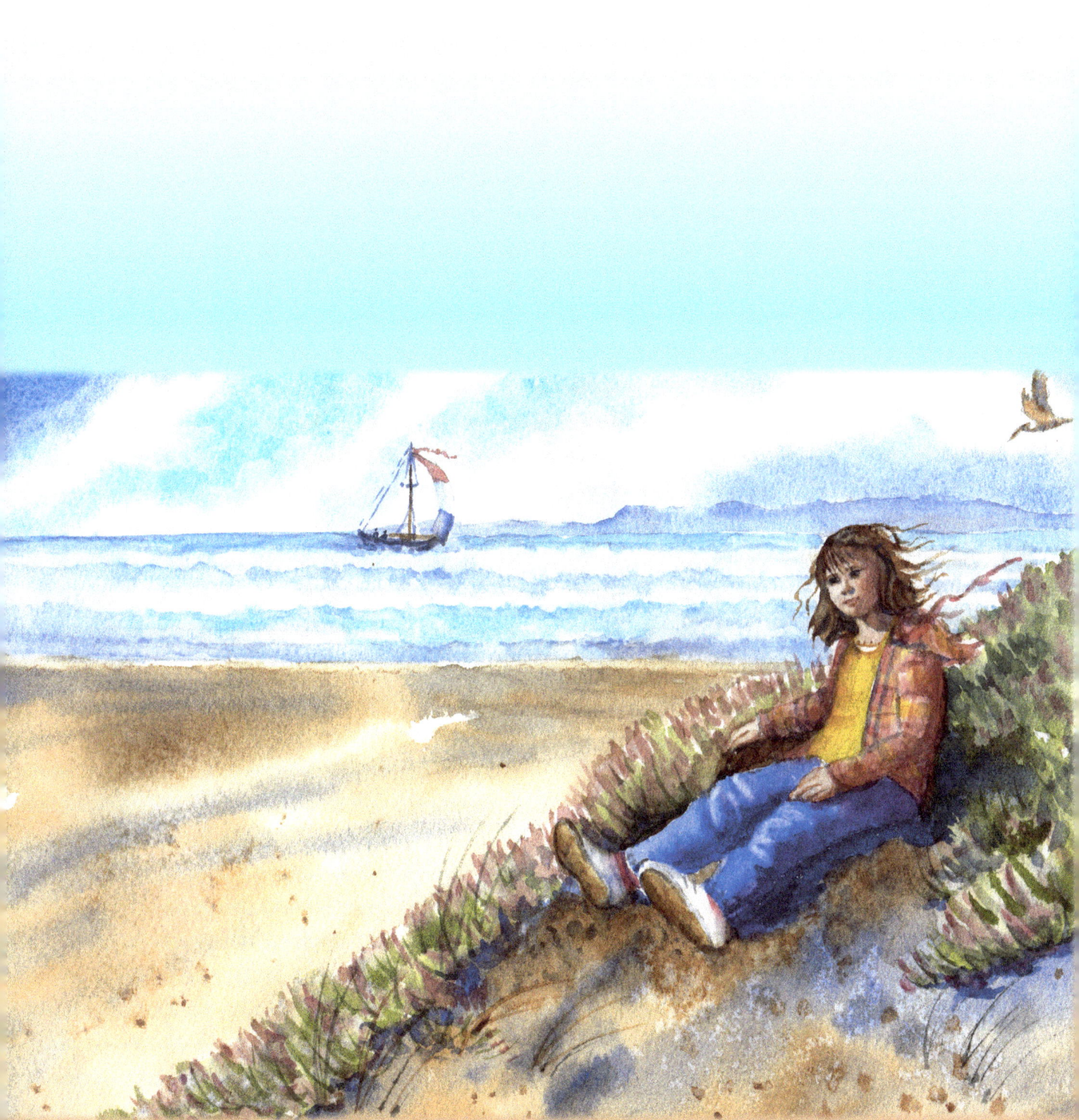

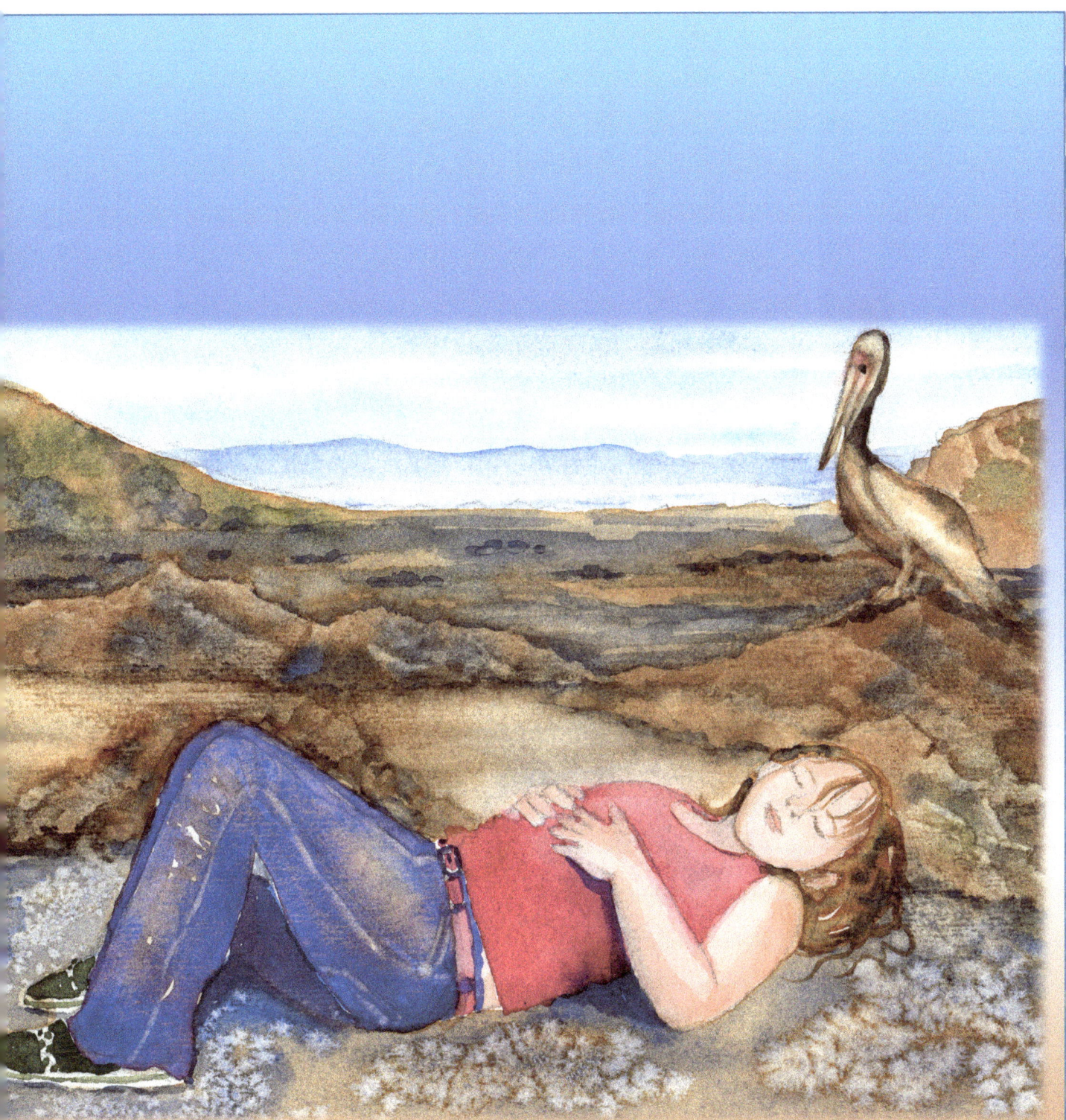

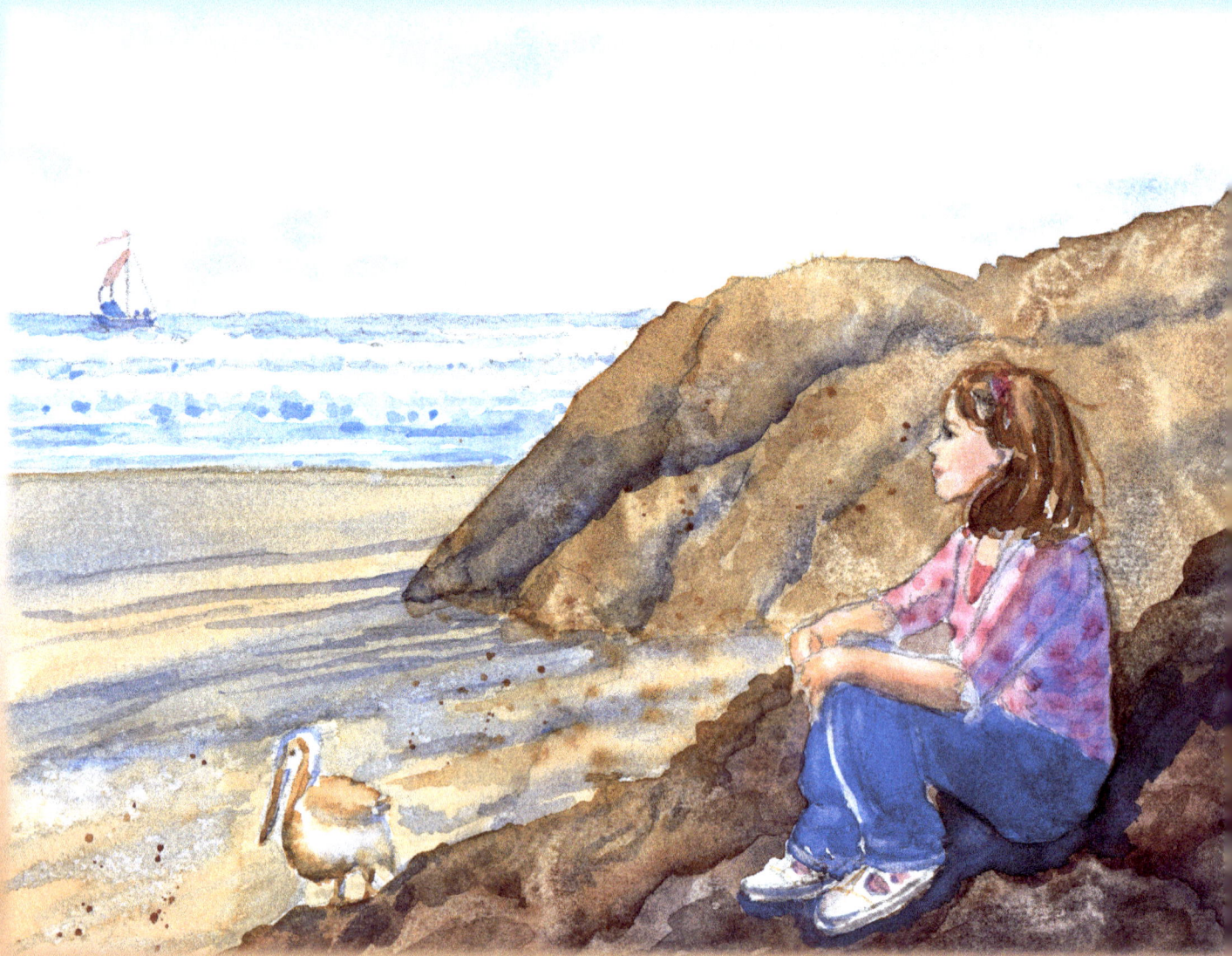

The Life In Me

Life is our most precious gift.
We are all connected to the family of living beings and to the circle of nature.
Our bodies follow the rhythms of nature,
just like the trees and hummingbirds do.
All energy of life flows in a wave pattern –
inhale–exhale, warm–cool, hungry–full, day–night, awake–asleep, like this:

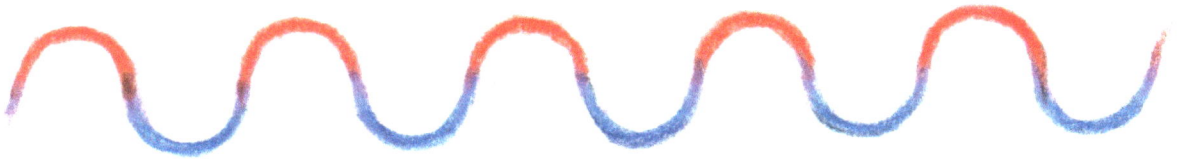

If we're rushed or bothered, the energy wave may go like this:

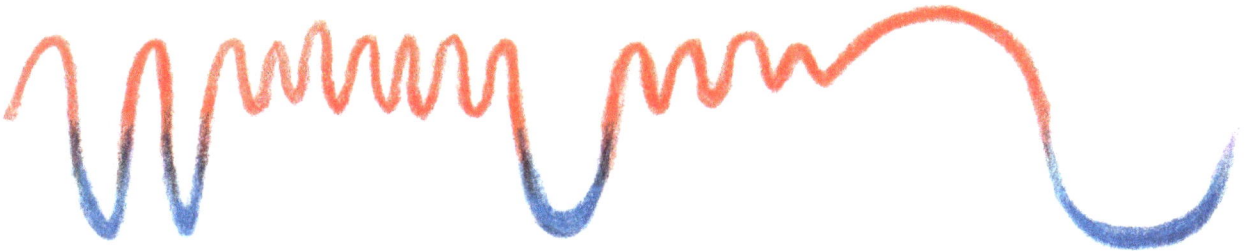

After being out of tune, we need some time for rest.
When the wave is gentle enough for us to heal,
we can come back to our usual energy wave:

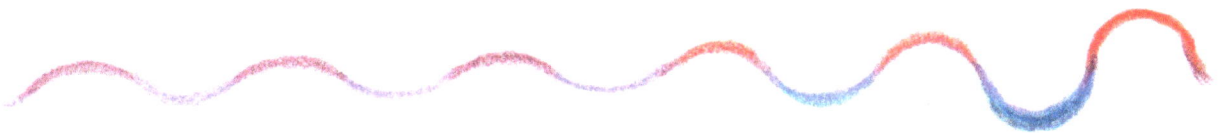

We are glad that our bodymind can ride the waves of life.
We can trust ourselves to heal.
We are thankful that our bodymind knows how to heal itself.
We can learn how to treat ourselves well and have lots of energy to play!

Diane Smalley, L.Ac., studied dance and theater from childhood through college, learning about the body from the inside. She began her acupuncture and herbal medicine practice in 1985. Soon after, she met C.W. Smith who taught her the basis of 'The Life In Me' series. Since then, she has been sharing these lessons with her clients, refining them. She has created a self-care curriculum for all ages, called "Seeds of Wellness." As we transition to more integrated health care, our contribution will be to accept more responsibility for our own health. Diane enjoys time in nature, design, dance and song.

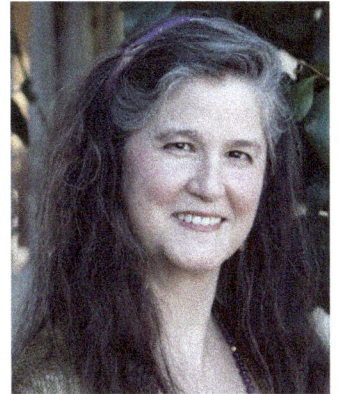

Ann Meyer Maglinte is the artist who created these exquisite watercolor paintings. One of Ann's first loves is watercolor. She has painted since she was a child, illustrating her own handmade books. Her paintings are in collections all over the world. She teaches at Mendocino College, and lives in a rambling home in the countryside of Willits. She has illustrated several books with pen & ink and watercolor, for adult fiction, field guides, and children's books. She is an herbalist, gardener, and enjoys choral singing.

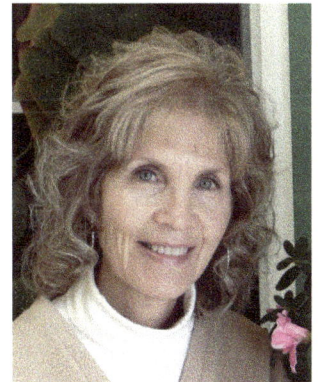

Explore The Life In Me series of books to expand your skill in self-care through fun and active stories.
TheLifeInMe.com
SeedsofWellness.co

ISBN 978-1-7326582-1-9